In memory of Nadezhda Lukianchenko.

Acknowledgments

Thanks to Julia Vlasova, for designing such a beautiful book, and to Jator Pierre for your creative input and for answering my endless list of questions; thanks to Scott Tenney at Blue Bird Canyon Farms for allowing me to work for a couple of months on your biodynamic farm in Laguna Beach. Thanks also to the following people for reviewing the material: Lisa Horgan, Alex Ravski, Eric Sung, Delini Malka Samarasinghe, Maxim Gantman, Kevin Merrell, Charles McGillivray, and Yi Liu.

The 1.5 Trillion Dollar Question...

"How did we survive 2.8 million years of evolution without doctors, therapists, nutritionist or medical drugs and have far better health (and vitality) then we do now?"
– Paul Chek

CONTENTS

Vegetables and fruits	6
Water	14
Eggs	21
Chicken	27
Beef	32
Fish	39
Pork	45
Turkey	51
Genetically modified food	56
Supplements	62
Is organic more expensive?	68
Biomagnification and toxic load	71

What this book is all about

    This book is designed to be an ABC guide for those looking to transition from factory-farmed food to organic and, hopefully one day, to biodynamic food. You'll receive a clear and easy-to-understand outline of how to look past all the misleading marketing and labelling. You'll understand exactly what you're getting in your food, how it's was produced, and how it's going to affect your health. After you're done with the book, you'll have a clear understanding of what separates factory-farmed food from organic food (it's not just the price), and you'll understand if that difference is something you will want to take into consideration.

  Here is a quick list of a few of the topics covered:
-The difference between cage-free, free-range, and pasture-raised eggs and meats.
-How genetically-modified food is in almost everything you eat, and how to avoid them.
-Why factory-farmed meats cause inflammation in your body.
-Why seeing "vegetarian fed" labels are actually a bad thing, even if it's also labeled "organic."
-Why food grown with pesticides are destroying your health and accelerating disease.
-Why farm-raised fish is poisonous.
-How to source the highest quality water.
-And much more...

  I mean to keep this book simple and to the point so you can spend less time reading and more time taking action and actually improving your health.

How to use this book

To enhance your learning, this book comes with free video instruction. Please email me a receipt of your purchase at etrufkin@gmail.com. After I receive a picture of your receipt, I will email you the associated videos. Text and video combined will help provide an enhanced learning experience, as well as give you the tools necessary to take action that will provide meaningful change.

I wish you the best in your pursuit of health and wellness. Don't demand change in the world; be the change you want to see in the world.

Breaking down the terminology

To make this book easier to understand, I use generic phrases. Here they are, and here is what they encompass:
-Factory-farm: Farming practices that rely on synthetic pesticides to grow their crops and various drugs to grow their meats, such as chicken, beef, and turkey. This category also includes intensive animal farming.
-Pesticides: This refers to the countless herbicides, insecticides, fungicides, etc. that are used to grow vegetables and fruits, or sprayed on animals.

Worst, Good, Best Categories

Most chapters are divided into three categories of quality to help you make informed decisions about the food you purchase: Worst, Good, and Best. Following the categories, I provide an outline on what the differences among the groups are; why those differences are important to consider; and an example of where to buy the best-category food group.

CHAPTER 1

VEGETABLES AND FRUITS

Topics Covered:

- Difference between factory-farmed, organic, and biodynamic vegetables and fruits.

- Amount of chemicals used in factory-farmed vegetables and fruits.

- Why washing vegetables and fruits do not get rid of pesticides.

- Best places to buy organic and biodynamic vegetables and fruits.

WORST CATEGORY:

FACTORY-FARMED

The amount of chemicals used in the production of factory-farmed fruits and vegetables are on another level. Just to keep it simple, let's look at the production cycle of factory-farmed tomatoes from Florida, and the amount of chemical warfare that has to happen to produce a handful of tomatoes.

Before planting tomato seeds, the ground is fumigated with a very dangerous chemical called methyl bromide. After that's done and everything in the soil has been killed, the tomato seeds are planted, and the production cycle begins. During this cycle, the tomatoes are bombarded with a myriad of dangerous synthetic pesticides until they're ready to be picked. Once picked, they're cleaned off with chlorine, which is another pesticide.

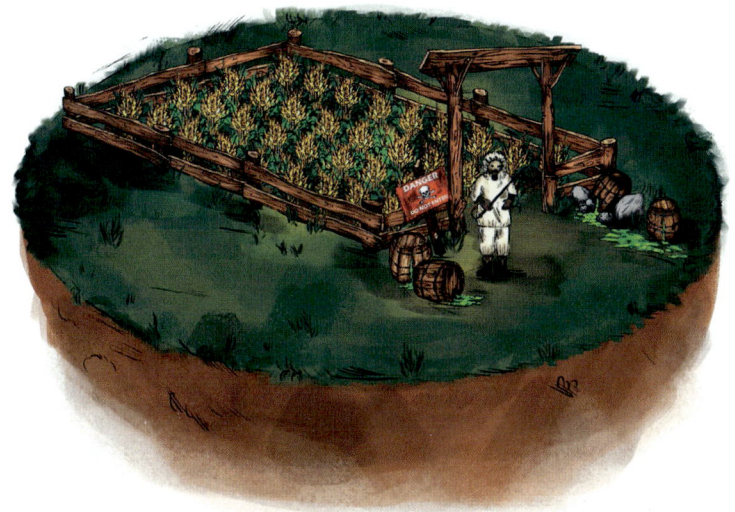

Once "clean," they're sprayed with an oil to give them a better look, and lastly, they are gassed with ethylene to help the tomato artificially ripen faster before they're shipped off to supermarkets. Those are a lot of chemicals!

And guess what? All these synthetic chemicals that are known to cause cancer, nervous system disorders, and birth defects don't just stay in the field. In fact, a large number of them are still found on your food when they reach the supermarket. In one investigation, the USDA reported pesticide residue in 85% of food tested.[1] Another study found that those eating a factory-farmed diet had pesticide concentrations in their system six times higher than those eating an organic diet.[2] Remember that pesticides are designed to harm the health of living organisms. People are living organisms.

Before we proceed, let's look at three common misconceptions regarding pesticide use on fruits and vegetables:

Misconception 1: Synthetic pesticides are tested for safety.

Common sense would have you presume that an entire chemical formulation is tested for safety before they are approved for use during food production. You would think that they would test entire chemical formulations in the lab to see if it contributes to various health problems; however, that's not what happens. In reality, chemical pesticides are composed of active and inactive ingredients, which are both listed on the back of labels. However, only active ingredients are required to be tested for safety, and not the entire formulation. Many of the inactive ingredients in a formulation, which could also add toxicity, are not required to be tested.[3] To summarize, an active ingredient in a specific chemical formulation could pass safety tests when tested without the presence of inactive ingredients whereas the entire formulation composed of both active and inactive ingredients may not pass the test. Often times, according to numerous studies, inactive ingredients increase the potency and potential toxicity of an active ingredient. Thus, a complete formulation may be more toxic than its active ingredient tested in isolation.[4]

Active ingredients tested in isolation pose problems. In reality, a myriad of pesticides is used in a single production cycle, as outlined above. Thus, most Americans could be exposed to trace amounts of numerous pesticides on a daily basis—not just one active ingredient of a single pesticide. A peer-reviewed study published by Dr. Theo Colborn, notes that "[i]t is fairly safe to say that every child conceived today in the Northern hemisphere is exposed to pesticides from conception throughout gestation and lactation regardless of where it is born."[5] Another study done by the Environmental Working Group found an average of 200 chemicals in newborns in America.[6] This is important to consider because it is obvious at this point that pesticides are making their way into the human body through the environment and through the consumption of food grown with such chemicals. Consequently, the more toxicity you have in your body, the more body fat your body has to create to store all these toxins. This is just one negative point. An increasingly serious problem is that these toxins end up lingering inside your body, thus increasing your body's toxic load, which could lead to all sorts of disease. According to the American Cancer Society, about 1/3 of Americans will develop cancer in their lifetime and half will die from it—could these pesticides be a cause?[7]

> ## Misconception 2:
> ## Pesticide residue found on produce isn't enough to harm one's health.

While some people recognize the presence of pesticide residue on their fruits and vegetables, they continue to presume that it's too insignificant of an amount to make an impact on their health. However, there are plenty of studies out there to prove otherwise. A study published in the peer-reviewed scientific journal Food and Chemical Toxicology found that levels of glyphosate typically found in humans, which was still below safety levels set by regulators, caused breast cancer cells to multiply.[8]

> ## Misconception 3:
> ## Pesticide residue can be washed off.

Remember that vegetables and fruit have roots that they use to absorb nutrients in order to grow. When you spray systemic pesticides on and around these plants, these pesticides go into the soil where they're absorbed by the roots of the plants. Once this happens, the pesticide becomes embedded in the edible flesh of the plant, which cannot be washed off. It is literally part of the whole plant at that point. Peeling the skin will also be ineffective because, again, the pesticide is embedded deep into the flesh of the plant. Every bite you take exposes you to this pesticide.

GOOD CATEGORY:

ORGANIC

The most common organic vegetables and fruits purchased are at the supermarket. Most organic vegetables and fruits found at the supermarket level are produced pretty much like a factory-farm operation, but with organic, or natural, means of pesticide reduction versus synthetic pesticides. If an organic crop of tomatoes were to be attacked by a hornworm, for example, the organic farmer would manually pick off the hornworm, whereas the factory farmer would just spray a bunch of chemical pesticides everywhere, killing the hornworm while simultaneously poisoning the soil and the tomato.

Other organic solutions to eliminate bugs that eat tomatoes would include yearly crop rotation, proper soil management, and the use of plant-based extracts and bacteria to organically control bugs. Sometimes predatory bugs are embedded to kill the hornworm without endangering the tomato. These are all examples of organic means used to get rid of bugs. Some supermarkets that sell large varieties of organic fruits and vegetables include Vons, Wholefoods, and Sprouts.

Alternatively, you can choose to purchase organic vegetables and fruits from a local, organic delivery service. Typically, these companies offer a monthly subscription to provide weekly home-delivery service of locally-grown, organic, and seasonal produce. It's important to know about the company and ask questions, but an example of one of these delivery services would be www.farmfreshtoyou.com. Farm Fresh to You is an organic farm co-op that's certified organic; they rotate their crops every single year, use organic means of controlling bugs, and only grow crops seasonally.

Another great option would be your local farmer's market. If you find the right organic farmer, this could be your best option in the entire category. A great farmer that's proud of their operation will always welcome you to come checkout their farm. Never be afraid to ask for a farm tour.

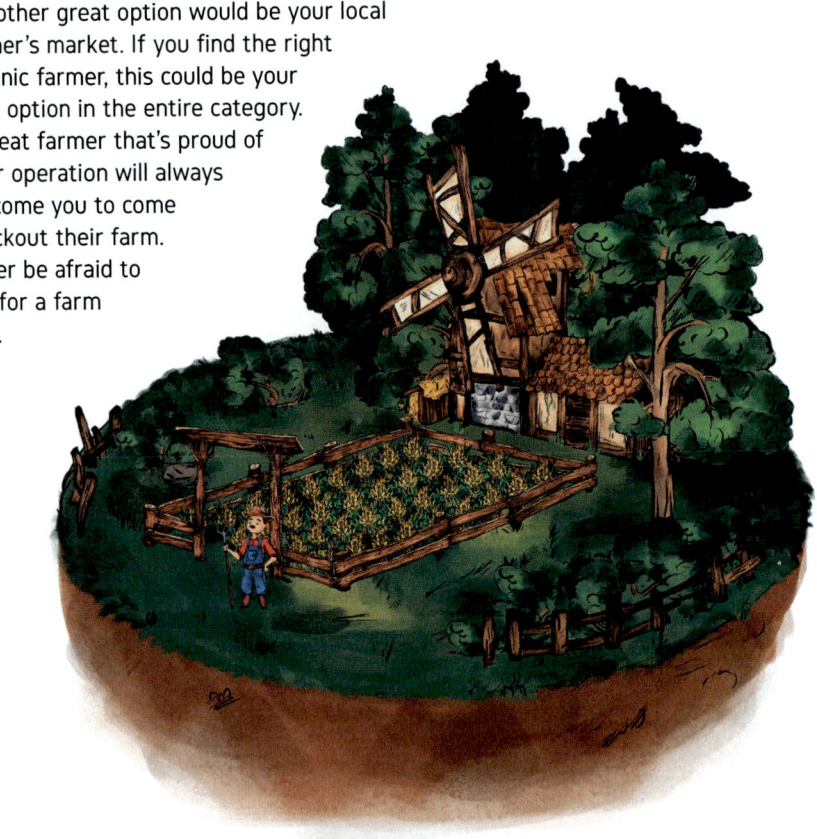

BEST CATEGORY:
BIODYNAMIC

Biodynamic farming is somewhat like the organic category above, except there is far more care and diligence put into maintaining soil health. They make sure to never take more from the soil than it can naturally produce. This seems like an insignificant difference, but it is actually very important to consider because everything you eat comes from the soil. If the soil isn't healthy, it will produce unhealthy vegetables and fruits, which you end up eating.

Another huge difference between biodynamic farming versus the two other categories is that biodynamic farming incorporates soil, plants, and animals into one self-sustaining system that tries to mimic nature as humanly possible.

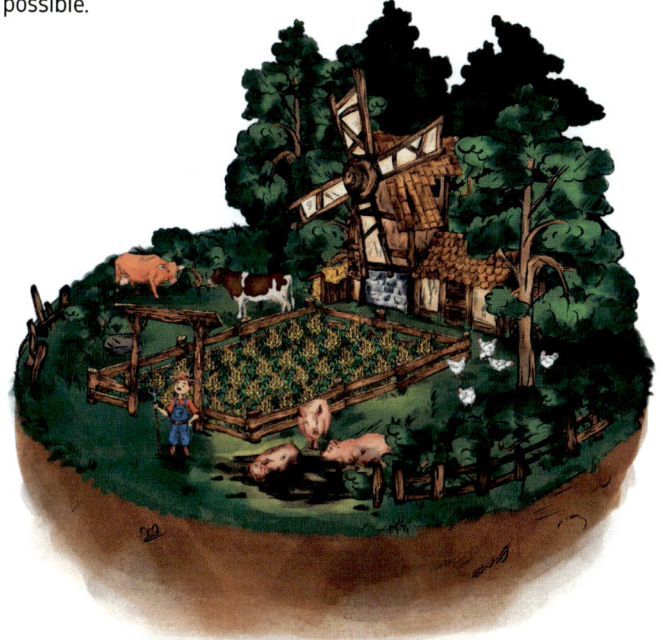

Nature is the best farmer around, so the closer you can get to producing food as nature does the better off you and your food will be. You won't see this type of holistic approach on organic farms typically, and you will never see it in the factory-farm category.

The best part of this is that biodynamic farmers are obsessed with soil health, fertility, and sustainability. Consequently, their plants that grow on their soil are healthy and strong. When plants are healthy and strong, pest infestations almost never happen. Remember that the role of pests is to kill off weak plants. Pests are basically nature's way of getting rid of weak plants, thus only allowing the strong plants to survive. If there are no weak plants, there are no pests, and thus no need for pesticides. If for some reason there is an outbreak, a biodynamic farmer would take a step back and focus on the health and the well-being of the entire farm as a whole. He would never resort to chemical pesticides like the factory farmer would. He would ask, "What's going on in the entire farm eco-system that would allow this tomato crop to be weak and unhealthy enough to be infested by hornworms?" Remember that pests, like hornworms, only exist when plants are weak enough to be attacked by them. No weak and unhealthy plants mean no bugs.

To remedy the situation, the biodynamic farmer would turn to boosting the health of the soil. Strong soil equals strong and healthy plants. He would, according to biodynamic farmer Ryan Goldsmith, "improve the soil microbiology by applying more farm-made compost, by applying herbal biodynamic preparations to the field, or some other seemingly indirectly applicable method that would benefit a particular aspect of the farm to boost its overall well-being." A good example of a biodynamic farm would be www.bluebirdcanyonfarms.com. Amish farms, as long as they have good biodiversity, could also be considered good examples of biodynamic farming. Also, although it's not 100% necessary, try to find farms that are certified through the Demeter Association (www.demeter-usa.org). Farms that are certified by the Demeter Association are far and few between, but if you have one in your area, more power to you.

Logos to Look for

At the supermarket level, the best possible combination of logos would be USDA Organic, Non-GMO Project Verified, and indication that the produce is locally grown. This combination of labels greatly decreases your exposure to pesticides and genetically-modified food. Since these vegetables and fruits are locally grown, they're fresher and they're produced in a more sustainable manner; moreover, you support your local community.

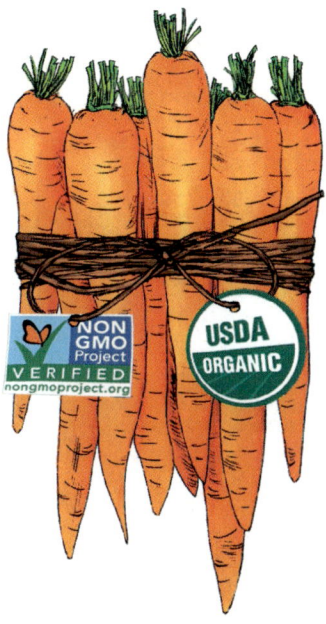

CHAPTER 2

WATER

Topics Covered:

- Difference among categories of water: distilled, reverse osmosis, tap, and artesian.

- How to objectively determine what healthy water is.

- How to determine if tap water is ideal to drink, and what type of filter is best for your tap.

- Water breweries and the life-giving force of artesian water.

Healthy water is dependent upon three variables:[1]

- The amount of hardness in the water.
- The amount of total dissolved solids in the water.
- The water's pH level.

- Hardness is defined by the amount of magnesium and calcium found in the water. The ideal hardness for drinking water is around 170ppm (part per million measured by CaCo3 – calcium carbonate). To determine if your water is of ideal hardness, purchase Hach Total Hardness Test Strips on Amazon.
- Total dissolved solids (TDS) is the total amount of inorganic and organic material found in water. The ideal TDS for drinking water is 300 ppm. To determine if your water has the ideal amount of TDS, purchase a TDS Meter with a digital aid on Amazon.
- Ph is basically a measure of how acidic or alkaline the water is. Ideally, you want the Ph to be at about 7.5 to 8, which means it's alkaline. To determine if your water has the ideal Ph, purchase Sanastec pH liquid drops, which are very inexpensive and can be found on Amazon as well.

WORST CATEGORY:

PURIFIED WATER

Water treated with a reverse-osmosis unit and distilled water should be avoided. At the supermarket, this type of water is typically sold as "purified water" or "distilled water," and is almost always sold in plastic—which is another negative. You want to avoid drinking water out of plastic at all times, because plastic increases the toxicity of the water, especially if left in the heat. Water that has been treated with reverse osmosis or distilled water has had every nutrient taken out of it, so you're basically drinking dead water. When I tested the Ph of various "purified" or "distilled" brands sold at the typical supermarket, they averaged out at a Ph of 3-4, which is very acidic. This type of water doesn't provide you with life, it takes life away from you.

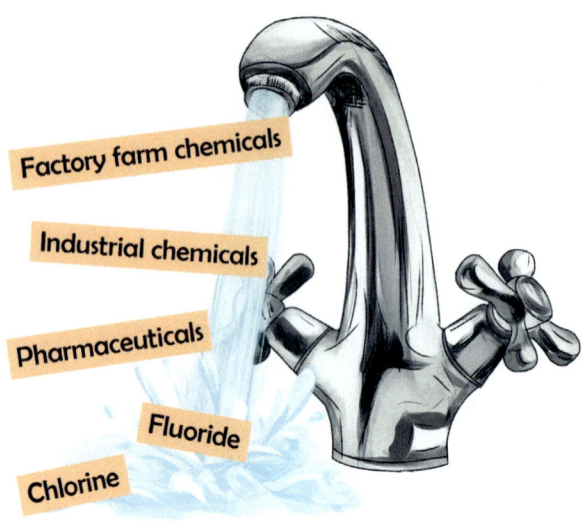

Another type of water to never drink is tap water without a proper filter. With the right filter, some tap water is actually great to drink and can easily be placed in the good or best category listed below. But to see if that's the case, lets run through a few steps and see if your tap water is good enough to drink.

First, determine if your tap water is ideal for drinking by using the three test kits listed above. If it's ideal, the next step is to test for which pollutants are present in your water.

As a general rule, it's important to know that water utility companies only filter out for major pollutants that will kill you or make you sick fairly quickly. They don't really do the best job at filtering out the little things that will harm your health long term. Knowing that, you have to understand that tap water has microscopic amounts of various pollutants and additives such as chlorine, fluoride, chemical run off from industrial plants, etc. Ideally, you want to filter these out of the drinking water as best as you can. Even small amounts add up overtime, especially if you're drinking water every day, as is ideal for health. Also, please remember that chlorine is a synthetic pesticide. You do not want that in your drinking water.

However, keep in mind that not all filters are the same. Some get rid of certain pollutants but not others. Don't presume that by purchasing just any filter will do. You have to purchase a filter that's specific to the pollutants in your specific area. Before determining which filter works best for your needs, you have to find out which pollutants and additives you're dealing with. Here are some easy ways to get that information:

Option 1

Your water utility company will post their water reports online. Simply find the website and download the forms from there. This report will give you an overview of various pollutants and additives found within your water. You can also call or email them and ask for the report to be mailed to you—which should be done for free. These reports are accurate enough. For my area, I hired a third-party company, and I tested the water myself. Both the third-party test and my own tests matched up fairly close to the results provided by the water utility company.

Option 2

Another option is to simply hire a third-party water testing laboratory. They're fairly inexpensive and will give you a good overview of what pollutants are in your water. I had a great experience with www.watersafetestkits.com

Once you determine which pollutants you're working with, it's time to buy the filter that is right for you.

One option is to do it yourself. In that case, a good book to checkout would be *The Drinking Water Book: How to Eliminate Harmful Toxins from Your Water* (2006) by Colin Ingram.

Another option is to take your water report to a local Home Depot and have an employee who understands water filtration systems pick one that's right for the type of pollutants you're dealing with.

Another option is to Google "water filter store near me" and go to one of those stores. Show them your report and go from there. I feel this is the best option.

The only disadvantage with filters is that as you filter out more and more pollutants, you also filter out all the minerals that your body needs to survive and thrive. And the more of those minerals you filter out, the less ideal the water becomes for your health. You want to be in the mindset of filtering as little as necessary, but at the same time keeping the pollutants out of the water as much as possible. It's a tough balance, especially these days.

Now that you have chosen your filter, it's time to test your water for hardness, TDS and Ph post filtration. It is this result that will determine if the water you are drinking at home is ideal for your health. Use your test kits to make sure the water's hardness, TDS, and Ph are ideal.

GOOD CATEGORY:

WATER BREWERIES

Water Breweries are companies that specialize in providing very clean water. Typically, they do a great job at reducing pollutants in the water and making sure the water has a great balance among the hardness, TDS, and Ph (the variables listed above). The only thing that sucks about water breweries, I feel, is that they typically filter their water via reverse osmosis. These systems are really good at getting rid of pretty much all pollutants in the water, but they also get rid of all the healthy, life-giving nutrients as well. They restructure and re-mineralize the water to bring it back to its natural balance, but I feel there are countless aspects of water we don't yet know how to scientifically measure, and these aspects, once destroyed through reverse osmosis, can in no way be reproduced through man-made efforts. An example of a water brewery would be www.thewaterbrewery.com.

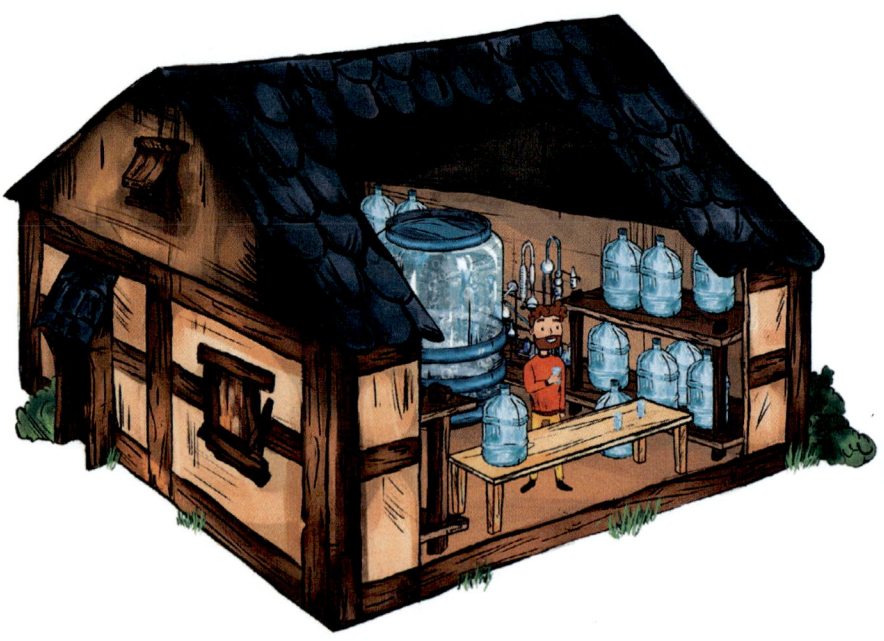

BEST CATEGORY:
ARTESIAN

Artesian water is actually a great source of natural water, which will provide you with an abundance of minerals in every glass at a perfect Ph. In my opinion, this is the best possible water you can drink. A site to checkout is www.findaspring.com. This site is great, and it will help locate artesian wells in your area. Fiji water is an example of artesian water that you can buy at a typical grocery store—although it's typically bottled in plastic. I'm using Fiji as an example because many people know about that brand, so they would understand what I'm referring to.

Mountain spring water bottled at the source in glass is another great option to choose from. www.mountainvalleyspring.com is a good example found in most stores. My all-time favorite would be Starkey Spring Water, which source their water from two miles deep within the earth and is bottled in glass. More information about them can be found at www.starkeywater.com.

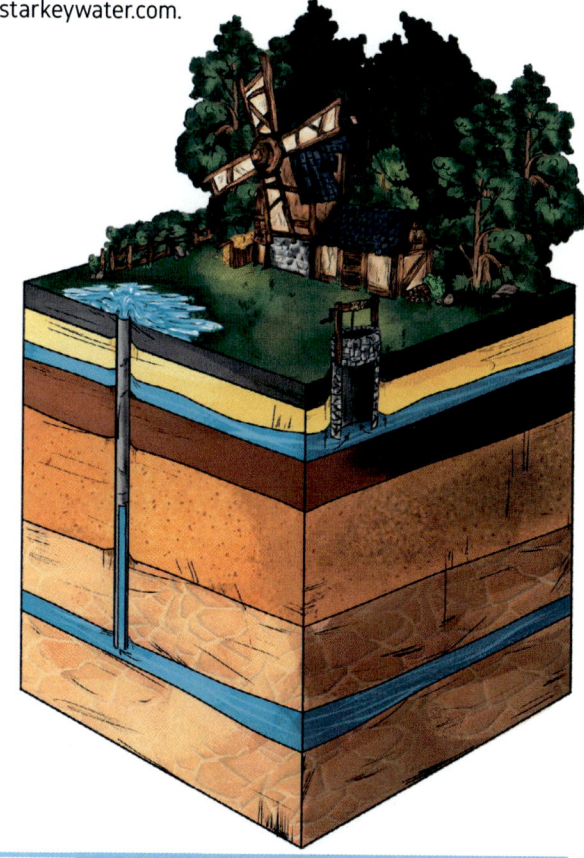

Tips to optimize your water

• If you're buying bottled water, purchase water that is bottled in glass.
• If you haven't turned on your faucet in twelve hours or so, make sure to run the water for 30 seconds before drinking. This will greatly help reduce the amount of lead and cadmium in the water you drink. The longer the water sits in the pipes, the more build-up of those heavy metals occur.
• Don't filter hot water. This will reduce the amount of contaminates the filter is able to remove. Filter only cold water.

Logos to Look for

A typical supermarket will have 10-15 different brands of water being sold on average. You want to seek out artesian water. It'll typically say "artesian water" right on the front. If it doesn't say artesian water, it's not.

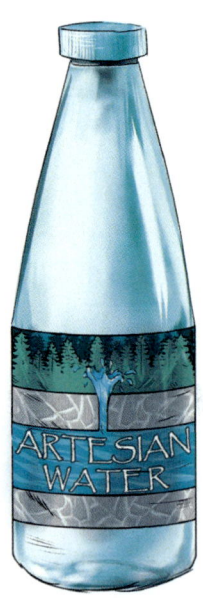

To get video instruction to this chapter, please email your receipt to etrufkin@gmail.com

CHAPTER 3

EGGS

Topics Covered:

- Difference between caged, cage-free, free-range, and pasture-raised eggs.

- Why "vegetarian fed" isn't a good thing.

- Why "free-range" and "cage-free" labels mean nothing.

- The importance of buying pasture-raised eggs.

WORST CATEGORY:

CAGED EGGS

Chickens raised in a *caged* environment are forced to live in horrible conditions. They literally spend their entire life in a cage no wider than a sheet of printing paper. Because of horrific conditions that lead to contamination, chickens in this category are constantly exposed to antibiotics because that's the only way to keep them alive in such a stressful and unsanitary environment. Just imagine being stuck with four human beings in a cage the dimensions of a queen-sized bed your entire life, and never being allowed to leave, stretch, shower, go to the bathroom in private etc.

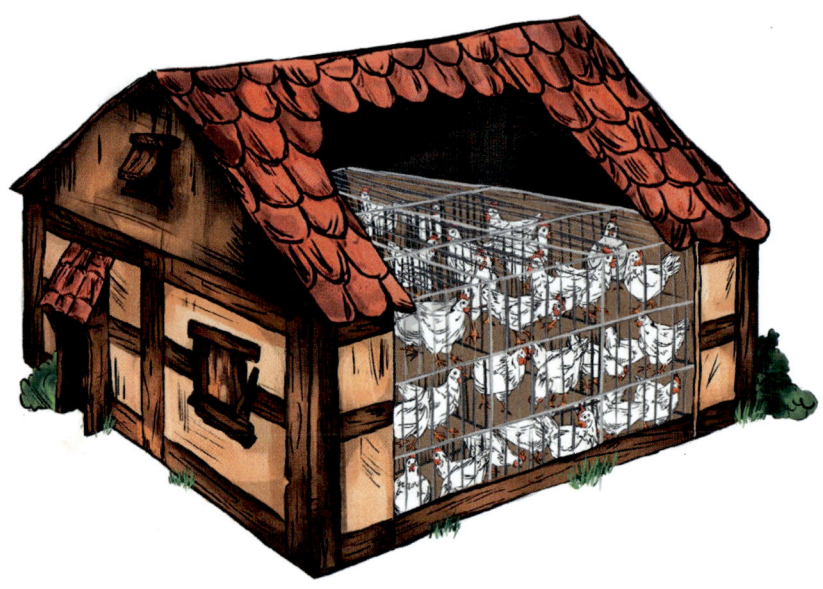

Another big negative is that most all of these operations rely heavily on feeding these chickens grains such as corn, which offsets the natural balance of omega-3 and omega-6.[1,2] Why is that important to consider? It's very important because if you're getting a tremendous amount of omega-6 in relation to omega-3 in your diet, the inflammation in your body is going to shoot through the roof.[3] According to Hunter, more inflammation means more joint pain, type 2 diabetes, fat gain, heart disease, Alzheimer's, cancer, depression, and the list goes on.[4]

Although it's a buck-fifty for a dozen eggs, I would highly recommend staying away from purchasing these eggs, and not only for your own personal health, but for ethical reasons as well.

Packages that don't state, "cage-free," "free-range," or "pasture-raised," are 100% caged eggs. Sometimes you will see "All Natural" or "Farm Fresh." This also indicates that the chickens are caged. Stay away!

BAD CATEGORY:

CAGE-FREE EGGS

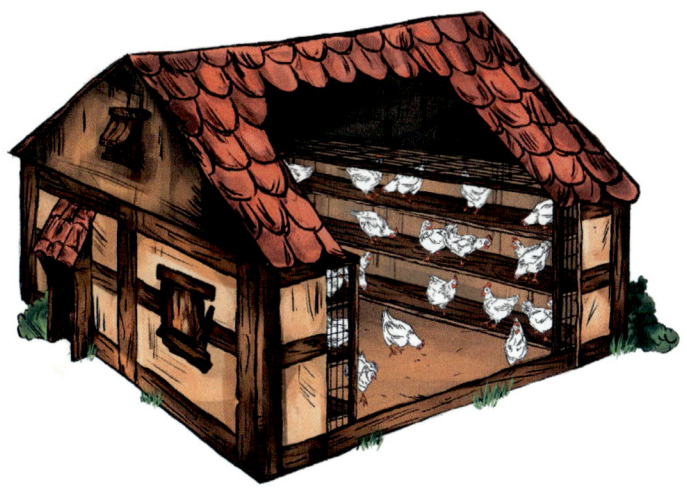

This is definitely heading in a better direction compared to "caged," but still bad. Here, the chickens aren't in a cage, but they get to roam around in a large, enclosed warehouse-type barn. However, it's still extremely cramped, and very unsanitary. Conditions, I would say, are still almost as terrible as the category above. Chickens never go outside, ever. The quality of egg is still not particularly good with this option because typically they're mostly all grain-fed chickens. If you see "vegetarian fed" on the label, that simply means they're most likely fed grain, such as corn. Chickens are naturally omnivores. They're supposed to eat an assortment of bugs and vegetables. They're not vegetarians! When you see "vegetarian fed" on the label, run! Once again, when they're fed grain, omega-6 shoots way up, which results in more inflammation in your body. Packages that state "cage-free," are in this category. I would stay away from this category, even if it's labeled "organic." If you see "cage-free" anywhere on the label, stay away. Run! Don't look back.

GOOD CATEGORY

FREE-RANGE EGGS

"Free-range" tend to be a fairly gimmicky phrase that doesn't mean much. Basically, in this category, you're still going to have a warehouse that's crammed tight with thousands of chickens. The only difference with this category versus the cage-free category mentioned above is that free-range chickens typically have a small concrete patio to hang out at during the day for a few hours here and there—maybe. Unfortunately, most don't even go outside. The doors leading to these patios are typically so small that most of the chickens don't even venture outside. So, at that point it's basically just the cage-free category above—with a slightly higher price tag. And once again, this category relies on grains such as corn as their main source of feed. You'll typically see "vegetarian fed" on labels sold as free-range chicken. That's actually not a good thing to see. It doesn't matter if it's organic. Organic grain is still grain. The balanced ratio of omega-6 to omega-3 is still destroyed, thus resulting in more inflammation.

What makes this operation "good" is because, on very few occasions, some companies do have a respectable free-range operation. But this is super rare, and most likely you will never see this at the supermarket level.

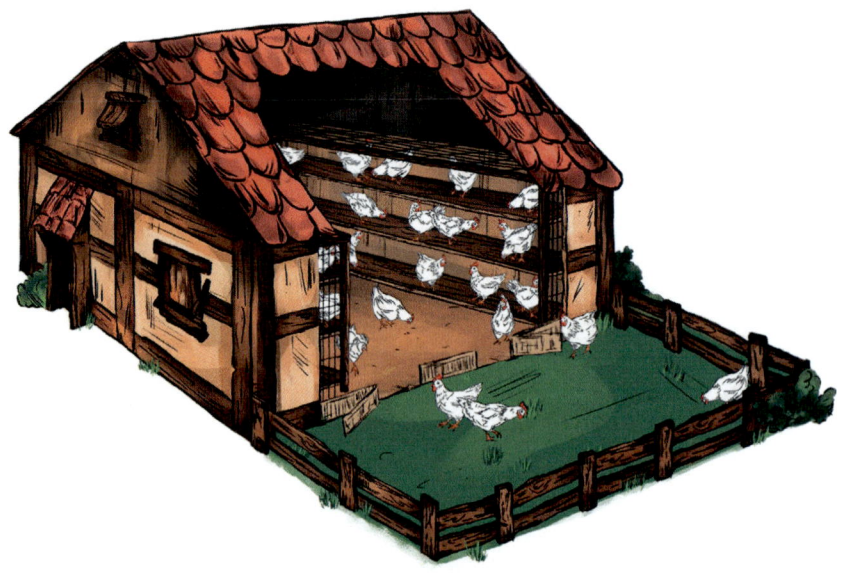

BEST CATEGORY

PASTURE-RAISED EGGS

If you're looking for chickens that roam on open pasture, enjoy the sunshine all day, have plenty of room to run around, and eat their natural diet of an assortment of bugs and greens, then you want to look for "pasture-raised" chickens. Pasture-raised chickens have healthier eggs. And because they're eating their natural diet, which includes bugs and worms, you'll get an ideal ratio of omega-3 to omega-6, and a lot more vitamin E and A than the three groups above. What does this all mean? This means way less inflammation in your body, which also means a healthier you.

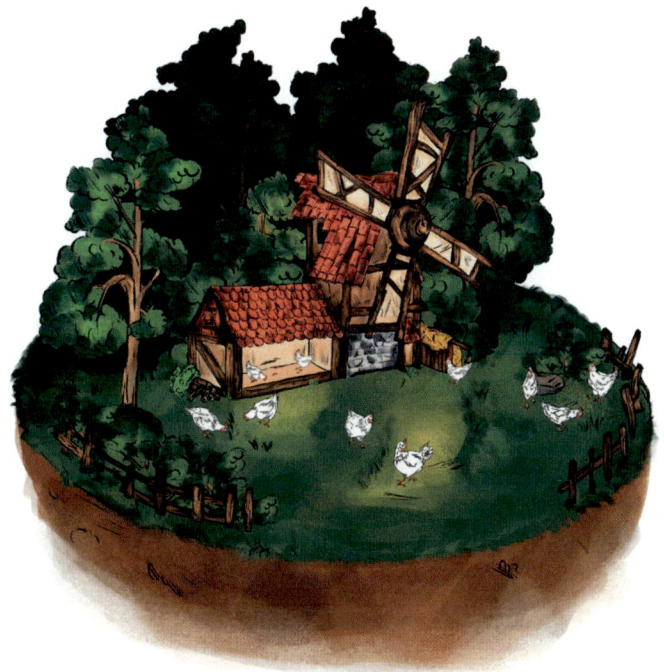

Although I'm sure many brands exist on the market, I like this brand of pasture-raised, USDA-organic eggs: Vital Farm's Pasture-Raised Organic Eggs. You can find these eggs at most supermarkets, especially at Sprouts and Wholefoods. Sometimes finding locally produced eggs is the best option. If you do find a local farmer that you want to buy from, ask the farmer if they comply with the following:
1. They grow their chickens in small numbers.
2. They don't feed their chickens corn or soy.

3. Their chicken feed is 100% organic.
4. They rotate the chicken onto new pasture regularly.
5. The chickens have 100-200 sq. ft of space per chicken.

Also, a legit farmer will always provide a free tour of their operation. Take advantage of this!

Logos to Look for

Buying quality eggs can be tricky. The best combination of logos to look for in this category would be "pasture-raised," "USDA Organic," "Min of 108 sq. ft (or above)," *and* corn- and soy-free. If they can top it off with locally grown, that would be the gold standard. An example of an amazing company would be www.happy-hens.com. You can also checkout a website called www.eatwild.com. Click on the "Shop for local grass meats, eggs and dairy" tab. After you select that tab, click on your state. Remember that most of these companies have home delivery options. If you definitely want to stick to the supermarket, go to www.cornucopia.org, click "score card", and then click "eggs".

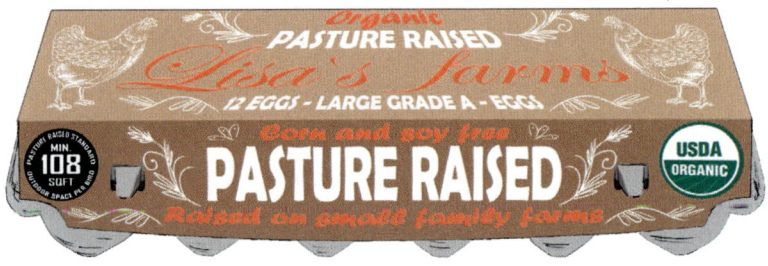

To get video instruction to this chapter, please email your receipt to etrufkin@gmail.com

CHAPTER 4

CHICKEN

Topics Covered:

- Difference between cage-free, free-range, and pasture-raised chickens.
- Chemicals found in factory-farmed chicken.
- Why pasture-raised chicken produces the healthiest meat.

WORST CATEGORY:

CAGE-FREE

"Cage-free" basically means that there are hundreds and thousands of chickens jammed into one warehouse building instead of a cage. They live shoulder to shoulder their entire life, and never, ever see daylight. They have almost no room to move at all, and they are drenched in their own feces and filth. Toxic ammonia and manure are everywhere. Over a six-week period, a single chicken produces 10 lbs. of feces. Multiply 10 lbs. of feces by the hundreds upon thousands of chickens jammed tight into these warehouses and you get a serious amount of feces and bacteria buildup that the chickens are constantly rolling around in all day. Maybe that's why a study done by the USDA "found that 87 percent of chicken carcasses tested positive for generic E. coli, a sign of fecal contamination, after chilling and just prior to packaging."[1]

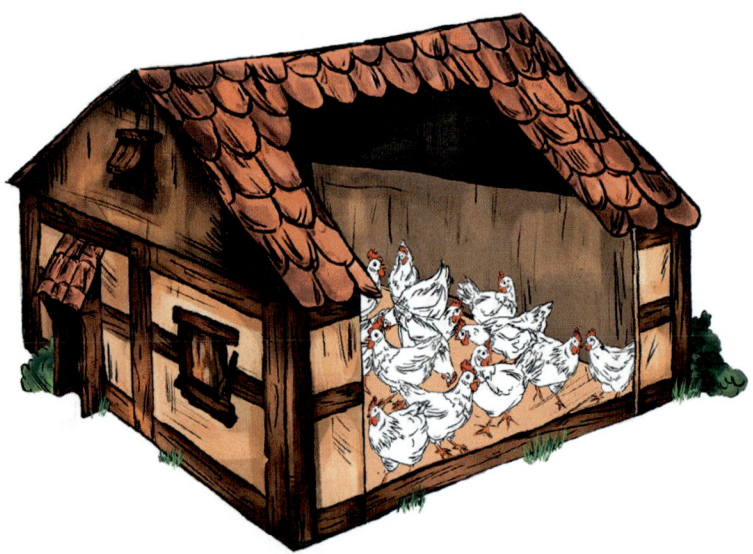

Because of these unsanitary conditions, which lead to a large number of chickens getting sick, the chickens have to be fed antibiotics regularly. According Mellon, Benbrook, & Benbrook, 75% of the nation's antibiotics are used in factory-farms, such as this cage-free category.[2] Since these antibiotics are used so often, they have become ineffective in maintaining chicken health, which results in forcing farmers to increase dosages in order for the antibiotics to work as they should.[3]

What else can be found in chicken sold from factory-farm operations? How about anti-depressants, Arsenic, banned anti-biotics, Tylenol, and Benadryl.[4] If you combine all the drugs, stress, and heavy reliance on grain feed, the nutritional profile of chickens in this category is very poor and toxic. Who knows what you're getting when you buy cage-free chicken? This is definitely a risk that should be avoided.

MODERATE CATEGORY:

FREE-RANGE

Free-range chicken is a step in the right direction, and the highest quality of chicken meat you'll find at your average supermarket; however, I'm not saying this is the best quality ever. This is just the best you'll get in the average American grocery store. Overall, I would rate this as "C"- level quality. What's different about free-range? Well, the warehouse is still jam-packed, just not as jam-packed as the category above. Also, the chickens get to roam outside in a small backyard, which is typically concrete, for a few hours per day. However, from my observation, the majority of chickens never actually go outside. Because thousands of chickens are concentrated in a small area, there are still tons of feces and bacteria everywhere. In my opinion, free-range at the supermarket level is a very gimmicky term, and it often means close to nothing. Most free-range chicken are also sold as "vegetarian fed," which is actually not a good thing to see on the label. Chickens aren't vegetarians; they're omnivores. They eat bugs and all sorts of other stuff. However, by "vegetarian fed," they mean grain fed! Grains drastically shoot up the omega-6, and thus offsetting the natural balance of omega-3 and omega-6, which results in more inflammation in your body.

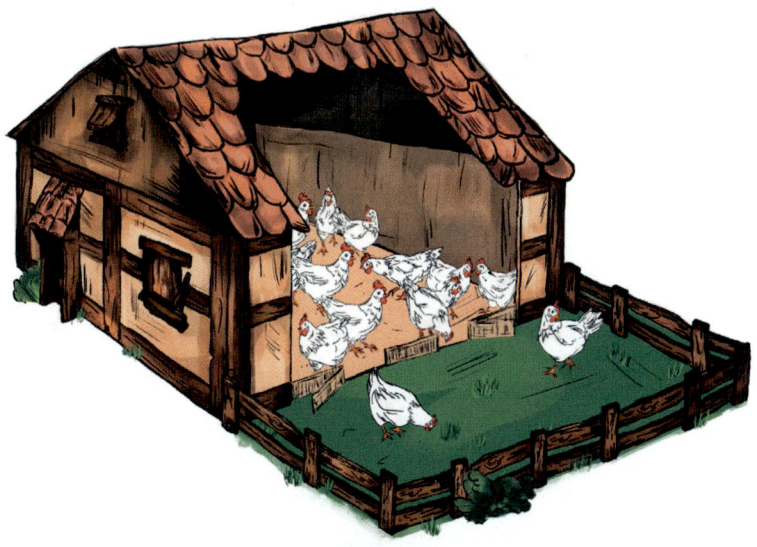

BEST CATEGORY:

PASTURE-RAISED

Here, the chickens get to roam on large, open farm lands their entire life. They have plenty of room to run around, and they get to hangout in the sun all day; they are social. They also eat a natural diet of various bugs and vegetables. Remember, chickens are omnivores. They're not vegetarians!!

Because of this natural, health-promoting environment, these chickens have great immune systems, which means the farmer doesn't have to use antibiotics. Their strong immune system will do the work just fine. An example of where you can buy pasture-raised chicken meat would be www.primalpastures.com. Wholefoods also sells pasture-raised chicken through Mary's Chicken. Just ask them for their "Step 5" pasture-raised chicken. You'll rarely find pasture-raised chicken sold in pieces. It'll only be sold as a whole chicken.

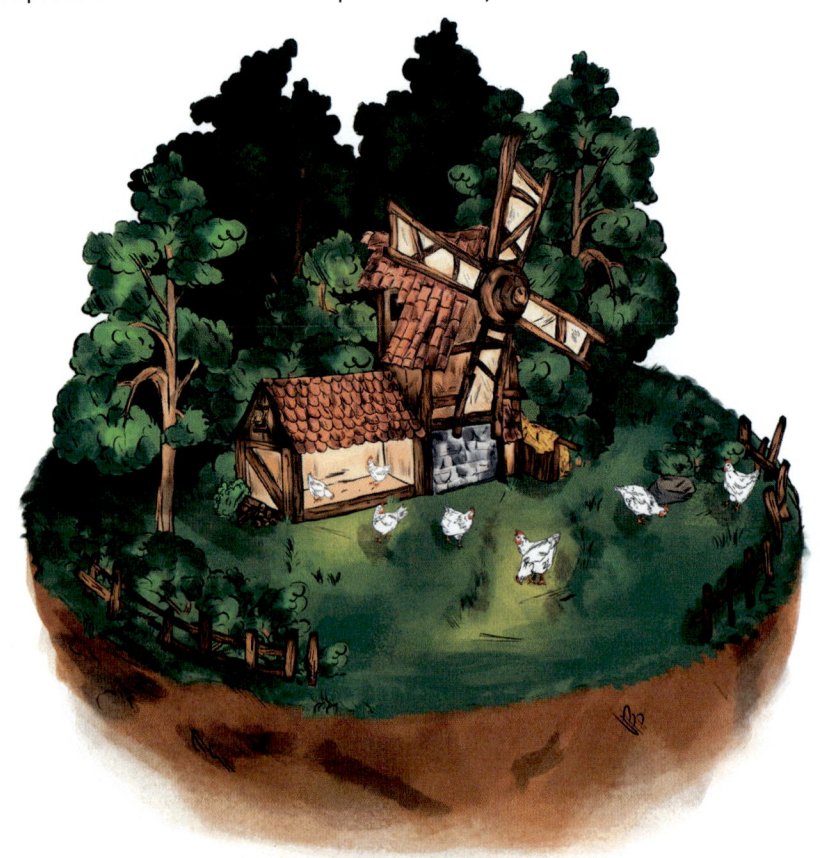

Logos to Look for

A good combination of labels to look for when buying chicken are "pasture-raised," "USDA Organic," "Non-GMO Project Verified" and "Locally Grown." If you see "Air Chilled" labels, that's also great, because it indicates a more sanitary processing method.

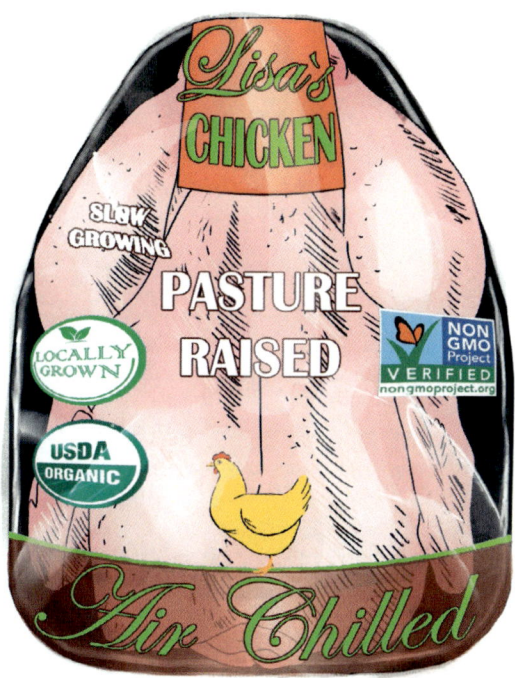

CHAPTER 5

BEEF

Topics Covered:

- Feedlot beef versus pasture-raised beef.

- Why feeding grain to cows is a bad idea.

- Chemicals used in feedlot beef.

- Where to buy 100% grass-fed, 100% pasture-raised, organic beef.

First and foremost, beef quality is basically divided into two categories. Before we go over those categories, it's important to understand that all cows raised for beef start off being raised on the pasture—not in a factory farm (feedlot). It's also important to understand that a cow's natural diet is mainly grass. They don't eat grains, because their body falls apart when they eat grains.

A few months before they're ready to be slaughtered and turned into the beef you see at the supermarket, 5% or so of the cattle remain on the pasture we mentioned before—mainly eating grass, their natural diet. However, 95% of the cows in America are sent to a feedlot for the remainder of their life. A "feedlot" is basically a factory-farm operation. Some are obviously managed better than others, but the general idea is that in feedlots, cattle are crammed into a pen, and they walk and lie in their own feces. They are usually fed grain not grass, and they are exposed to a myriad of antibiotics, sex hormones, and beta-agonist. Typically, it's these feedlot operations that give the beef industry a bad name.

WORST CATEGORY:

FEEDLOT BEEF

This category is all about high-volume, low-quality beef. The cattle in this category are raised on sex hormones, antibiotics, beta-agonists, industrial byproducts, and grain, which usually come from genetically modified sources grown with harmful, synthetic pesticides. You think all those chemicals don't make their way into the meat fibers and fat of the beef that you end up eating?

Think again.

One study compared beef from Japan, where the use of sex hormones is illegal, to beef from the United States, where the majority of cows grown for beef are exposed to a cocktail of various sex hormones and it's totally 100% legal. Researchers concluded that U.S. beef had around 600 times more estrogen then beef from Japan.[1] Why should you care?

It matters because a high concentration of estrogen in the body leads to the following side effects: increased fat around the chest for males, loss of muscle tone, decreased sex drive, erectile dysfunction, and an increase in estrogen-dependent cancers, among other things.

To add insult to injury, in 2010, the Food Safety and Inspection Services discovered that hundreds of cows sent to slaughter for beef had illegal amounts of drug residue in their organs, and this wasn't a short list of drugs either. And yes, these products ended up in the grocery stores you frequent. The investigation found the following drugs: penicillin, flunixin, sulfadimethoxine, gentamicin, sulfamethazine, tilmicosin, and ampicillin. Gentamicin remains in the animal's system for up to three years.[2]

On top of all the drug use, another issue with feedlot beef is that they feed the cows heavy amounts of grain, which destroys the natural omega-3 to omega-6 ratio, resulting in more inflammation in those who consume the meat. In this category, you'll also see less CLA, vitamin-E, beta-carotene, calcium, magnesium, potassium, B vitamins, and riboflavin.[3]

I would stay away from this category simply to reduce your exposure to sex hormones and various other drugs administered to the cattle. The omega-3 to omega-6 ratio is also terrible, which could lead to inflammation that creates a lot of problems in your body and mind.

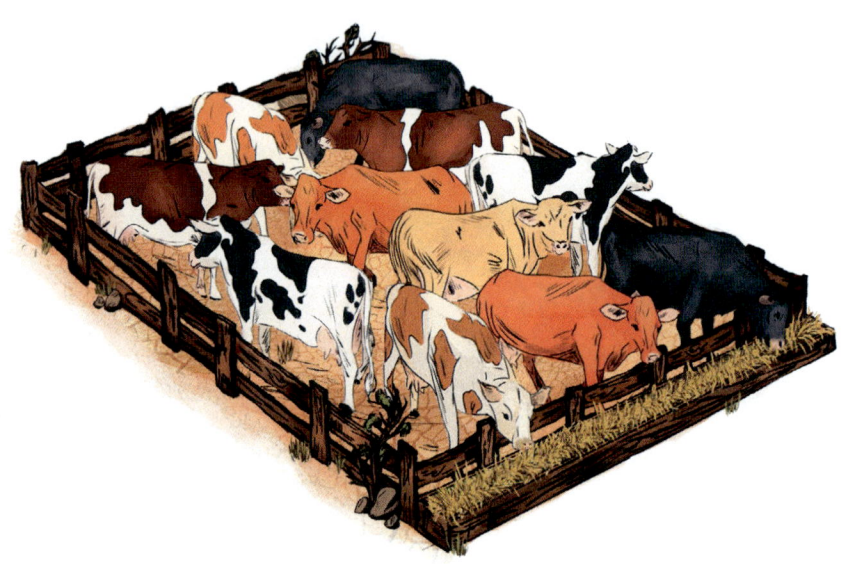

BEEF

BEST CATEGORY:

PASTURE-RAISED BEEF AND 100% GRASS FED

This is the best possible category of beef you can buy. Typically, this category is 100% pasture-raised, 100% grass fed, and 100% organic. What does this mean? Well, this means NO exposure to synthetic sex hormones, antibiotics, GMOs, beta-agonists, synthetic fertilizers, or pesticides, etc. This is the cleanest possible category of beef.

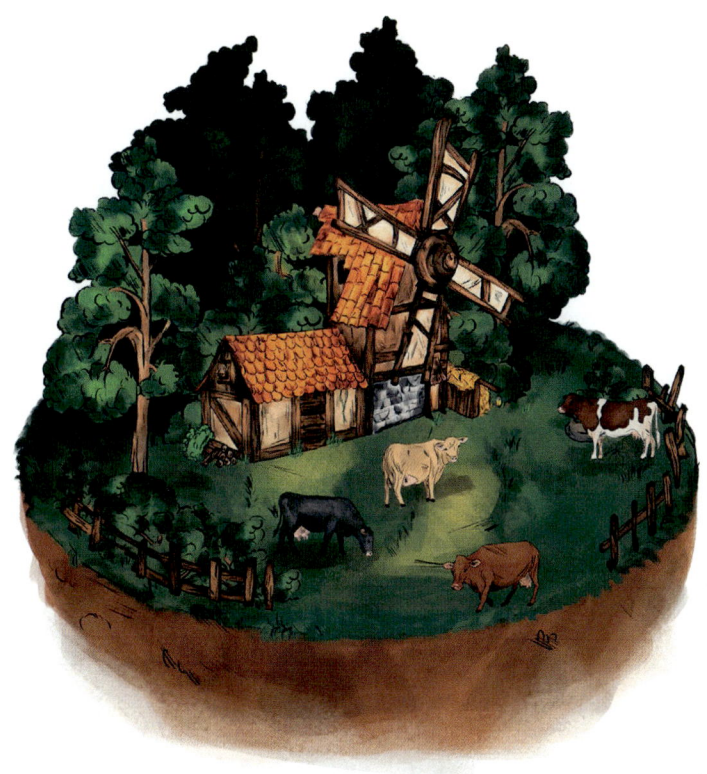

On top of that, since this beef is 100% grass-fed, their nutritional profile is going to be the best out of the categories listed here. You'll get a good dose of omega-3, CLA, iron, vitamin E, a bunch of vitamin B, and a good amount of riboflavin. Plus, since these cows are not fed grain, the ratio of omega-3 to omega-6 is great and very health promoting.

You can typically find beef of this category at places like Wholefoods and Sprouts. At Wholefoods, look for Eel River Organic beef (www.certified-organic-beef.com). For Sprouts, look for 100% grass-fed beef that's organic. Once again, it must say both "100% grass fed" *and* "Organic."

Also, you can find a small local farmer like www.primalpastures.com. Their beef is 100% grass-fed, 100% pasture-raised, and never supplemented with genetically-modified feed. Their beef is also organic, which means they don't use steroids or antibiotics. They also have a delivery service and offer free farm tours.

Ground-Beef Warning

95% or more of ground beef comes from older, worn-out dairy cows (cows used for milk and milk products). These poor animals have been forced to live their entire lives in extreme confinement. They are also continuously artificially impregnated in order to produce milk all year round. They are also exposed to a myriad of drugs to keep them from dying (the conditions in these confined operations are terrible). Also, ground beef is composed of numerous pieces of different dairy cows, so the chances of cross-contamination is higher.

Prentice (2011) noted that "According to the FDA, while 7.7 percent of cattle slaughtered in the United States are dairy cattle, a disproportional 67 percent of drug residue violations are tied directly to dairy cattle." If you do get ground beef, I would recommend that you definitely buy organic and definitely make sure it has a "100% grass-fed" label. Visit the farm if you can. If a farmer refuses to give you a tour, do not buy their products. The refusal to give a farm tour is a huge red flag. A farmer who is proud of their operation and has nothing to hide will always happily give you a tour. End of story. One of the common excuses a shady farmer will give when refusing to provide a farm tour is this: "we try to keep the animals healthy by not exposing them to outside guests." I've heard this one so many times in the past, and it is completely false. Let the farmer know that they are clearly hiding something and don't buy from them.

"Prime," "Select," and "Choice" labeling confusion

Often times on packages of beef you'll see "USDA Prime," "USDA Select," and "USDA Choice." This is basically a rating system for how much fat is found in the product. "USDA Prime" is given to cuts that have the highest amount of fat. This is actually not a good thing, especially if the beef isn't organic and it is fed grain. Remember that toxic chemicals are stored in fat. Thus, the more fat content in the product means the more toxic chemicals, and USDA prime cuts have the most amount of fat. People often buy beef with the "USDA Prime" label thinking they're getting an awesome deal because it's more expensive and says, "USDA Prime." In reality it's the complete opposite. Stay away from USDA Prime and understand that it's not a symbol of quality. Don't be fooled by the label.

Kobe Beef Warning

Kobe beef is probably one of the worst beef products you can buy on the market. This beef is basically grain-finished beef. Like I mentioned above, that means the natural omega-3 to omega-6 ratio is destroyed, thus causing a tremendous amount of inflammation in those who consume it. I know Kobe beef is expensive, but I honestly don't know why. Personally, I wouldn't buy Kobe beef, ever.

"Grass Fed" VS. "100% Grass Fed" confusion

Sometimes you'll see labels that claim their beef is grass fed, which isn't a lie, but is somewhat misleading. Since all cows raised for meat are raised on pasture for the majority of their life, all beef could be considered grass fed. But remember that the majority of cows start their life on pasture eating grass, but then a minimum of 95 percent, and sometimes more, are sent to a feedlot where they're all fed heavy amounts of grains for a few months before they're killed. Those short few months where the cows are fed grains (which, again, is not their natural diet) changes the nutritional profile of the beef significantly, and not for the better.[4] Thus, the cows that start on pasture but are sent to feedlots are considered "grass fed" and "grain finished." The other 5% that never left the pasture and that you want to buy are considered "grass fed" and "grass finished," or "100% grass fed." Go for the 100% grass-fed beef. Avoid grain finished, feedlot, factory farmed beef.

And make sure it's organic. On the packaging, look for things like "organic," "certified organic," or "USDA organic." These are all indications that it's organic. Another thing you can do is look for grass-fed beef that's certified through www.americangrassfed.org. In fact, at the bottom of their website, you'll see an interactive map. Go to the map, click on your state, and find a legit grass-fed operation near you. I buy mine from www.5barbeef.com and www.azgrassraisedbeef.com. Another great company to checkout would be www.primalpastures.com.

Logos to Look for

When seeking out beef, make sure you see "USDA Organic" and "100% grass fed." Seeing these two together are key indicators of high-quality beef. Don't fall for "Product of the USA" labeling claim. A beef carcass can be shipped from Mexico, cut up and packaged in the USA, and labeled "Product of the USA". This is important to consider because the U.S. imports the bulk majority of its grass-fed beef. Once again, another thing you can do is make sure they're certified through www.americangrassfed.org. If they are, that's always a good sign. Remember, most of these farms offer home delivery service. Organ meats are always the cheapest and actually the most nutritious.

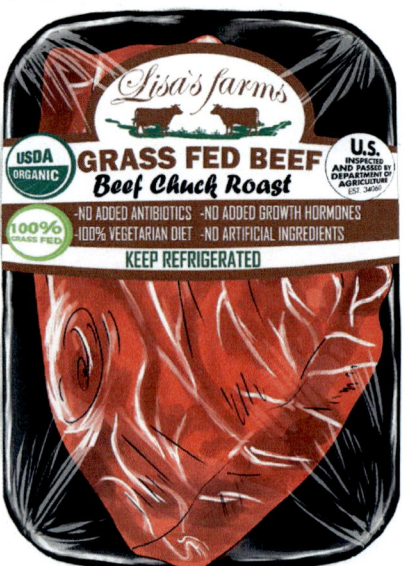

To get video instruction to this chapter, please email your receipt to etrufkin@gmail.com

CHAPTER 6

FISH

Topics Covered:

- Difference between farmed-raised fish and wild-caught fish.
- Toxicity of feed given to farm-raised fish.
- Pesticides used in farm-raised fish.
- Ocean toxicity and how to avoid mercury in wild-caught fish.
- Which species of fish are the best to buy?
- Where to buy the best wild-caught fish.
- Should I buy frozen or fresh fish?

WORST CATEGORY:
FARMED FISH

Just like any factory-farm operation, which this category is, you'll see a lot of confinement. In a factory-farm operation, you'll see maybe hundreds and thousands, or even millions of fish, and this is called aquaculture. These fish factory farms could be found on land, on the coast, or sometimes even out at sea—always in cages, of course.

Because these operations stuff so many fish into a small, enclosed area, diseases constantly break out—just like any factory-farm operation. To combat them, farmed fish operations would regularly implement industrial amounts of antibiotics, as well as very toxic synthetic pesticides.

To make matters worse, farmed fish are also fed very toxic, low-quality feed, which typically have a laundry-list of chemicals such as PCBS, Dioxin, and ethoxyquin.[1,2]

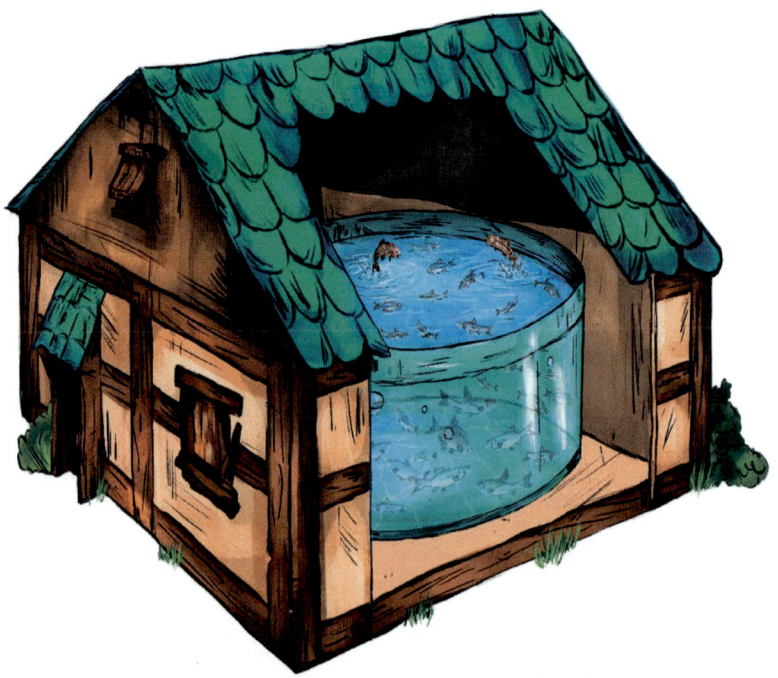

Once the farmed fish eat this feed, the chemicals are absorbed into the tissue of the fish, which gets passed down to the consumer. One study found that 96% of tested farmed fish samples had traceable amounts of ethoxyquin, some samples having 10-20 times the permissible amount in other food products. Whereas in the same study, wild-caught fish had no traceable amounts.[3] I know there is a lot of talk about antibiotics used in food production, but it's important to understand that this feed and the chemicals present in it are even more dangerous for your health than exposure to trace amounts of antibiotics through food. Extremely low levels of these chemicals can have a negative effect on your hormonal system; moreover, it can possibly lead to cancer.

Another drawback of feeding the fish poor quality feed (dried protein and/or genetically modified corn/soy pellets) and having them live in an unnatural, confined, and stressful environment is that they throw off the omega-3 to omega-6 ratio. You typically find a really high level of omega-6 in farmed fish, but very little omega-3, which again contributes to inflammation and disease in those who eat this category of fish. On the package, if you see things like "Atlantic Salmon," "tilapia," or "farmed fish," that means it's most likely from this category. The majority of shrimp sold at the supermarket are also farmed. Look for the label. Stay away at all costs.

BEST CATEGORY:

WILD-CAUGHT FISH

No matter how you cut it, wild-caught fish will have a far better nutrition profile and far less toxicity than their farmed counterparts. As I've mentioned, wild-caught fish are far less toxic than farm-raised fish. However, because the world's water these days is contaminated with mercury and other harmful contaminates, to be safe you have to choose wild-caught fish based on the following 3 criteria: mercury to selenium ratio, location the fish is caught, and nutritional value.

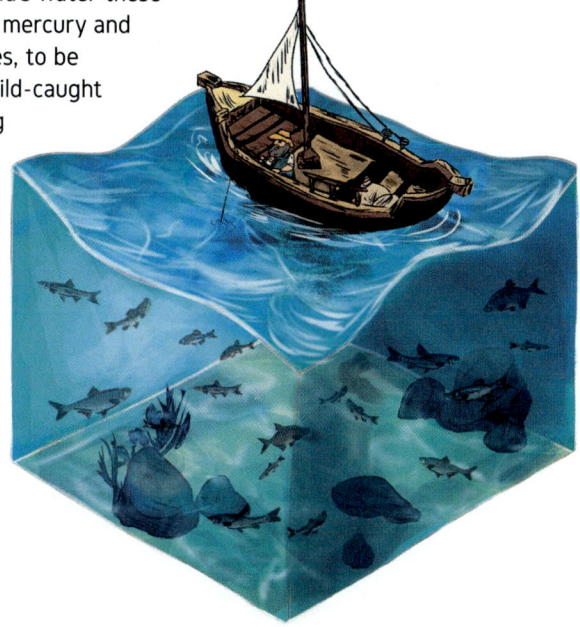

Mercury

Mercury is considered one of the most dangerous chemicals circulating in the environment, and it is a byproduct of industrial operations—mainly from burning coal. Once mercury gets into the ocean, it is converted into methylmercury, where it makes its way into the food chain. It is basically present in every single fish you find out at sea, but to varying amounts depending on the fish. Methylmercury is toxic. However, you can easily avoid the negative health effects of mercury by simply buying fish that are low in methylmercury and have an ideal selenium to methylmercury ratio. Ideally, you want higher selenium to very little methylmercury.[4, 5]

Location

Unfortunately, mercury isn't the only chemical polluting the oceans; there are a number of pollutants in the water depending on location. There are a number of heavy metals, radioactivity from nuclear weapons testing, disasters like Fukushima, micro-plastics, petrochemicals from oil spills, pharmaceutical drugs (which are discharged into the ocean), and contaminates from factory-farming and industrial plants. All of these contaminates add to the overall toxicity of the ocean's water; thus, a lot of these contaminates can be found in varying degrees in the flesh, organs and fat of wild-caught fish. Thus, it's important to know where the fish you're buying comes from and what contaminates are present in that area. Personally, I just buy wild-caught fish from Alaska.

Nutritional value

The biggest advantage of eating fish over all other types of proteins is the large amount of bioavailable omega-3 fatty acids you would get from the fish. Vegetables may have omega-3, but the absorption is very poor. Land-based animals, such as 100% grass-fed beef, also have omega-3s, and although more available, the amount is small when compared to what you would get in wild-caught salmon, or sardines, for instance.

Here are some examples of the ideal fish you could be buying, which take into account the three variables mentioned above:
•Wild Alaskan Sockeye salmon, silver Salmon, and Artic Keta Salmon

- Wild Alaskan Cod
- Wild Alaskan Sablefish (Black Cod)
- Wild Alaskan Halibut
- Sardines from Canada or USA either bought fresh or packed in water or organic olive oil

Purchasing instruction

Fresh Vs. Frozen:
I personally buy frozen fish over fresh supermarket fish out on display. It's one thing if the fish you bought was caught that same morning, but most of the time the "fresh" fish you see displayed at the supermarket is possibly a few days to a week old. That means that fish has been laying out and decaying for maybe seven or more days. That's just way too long. It's not considered very fresh at that point. Choose frozen fish instead. It'll actually be "fresher," and the nutritional profile will also be better because it won't be so decayed.

Where to buy:
You can find most of the fish I have listed above at Wholefoods or Sprouts. However, the only company I've been able to find that offers high-quality fish in the USA is https://www.vitalchoice.com. From my research, Vital Choice gets a lot of their fish from Alaska, and from areas that have not been exposed to large amounts of pesticides, dioxins, organobromides, and furans. Vital Choice selects species that aren't likely to carry persistent organic pollutants, and they don't overfish.

Logos to Look for

Don't fall for the Atlantic Salmon marketing scam. Whenever you see "Atlantic Salmon," that means farm-raised and not wild-caught. What you want to see on the label is "Wild-Caught" fish. If it doesn't say that, it is farm raised.

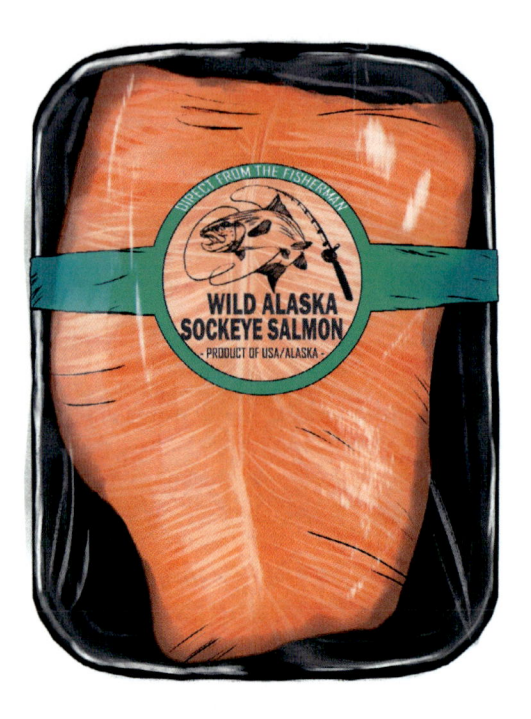

CHAPTER 7

PORK

Topics Covered:

- Difference between factory-farm, free-range, and pasture-raised pork.
- Why you should worry about the secret drugs used in factory-farmed pork.
- Supermarkets only sell factory-farmed pork.
- Where to buy pasture-raised pork.
- Why feeding pigs grain is bad.

WORST CATEGORY:
FACTORY-FARM PORK

Sadly, the majority of pork sold in supermarkets come from a factory farm. In fact, I couldn't find a single supermarket that purchased pork from non-factory farm operations. These operations produce pork inhumanely; and, as we've learned earlier, inhumane treatment and production of pork often means that the quality of the meat is sacrificed. To understand what I'm getting at, lets walk through the step-by-step process of producing pork at a factory farm.

First, the female pig is artificially impregnated and then confined to live in a cage for the duration of her pregnancy, which is four months. This cage gives her just enough room to stand up and to sit down. There is literally not enough room to even turn around. To make things worse, she's never allowed to leave her cage, nor is she exposed to natural sunlight; instead, she lives her entire life under artificial lights. Moreover, she is forced to live in her own urine and feces.

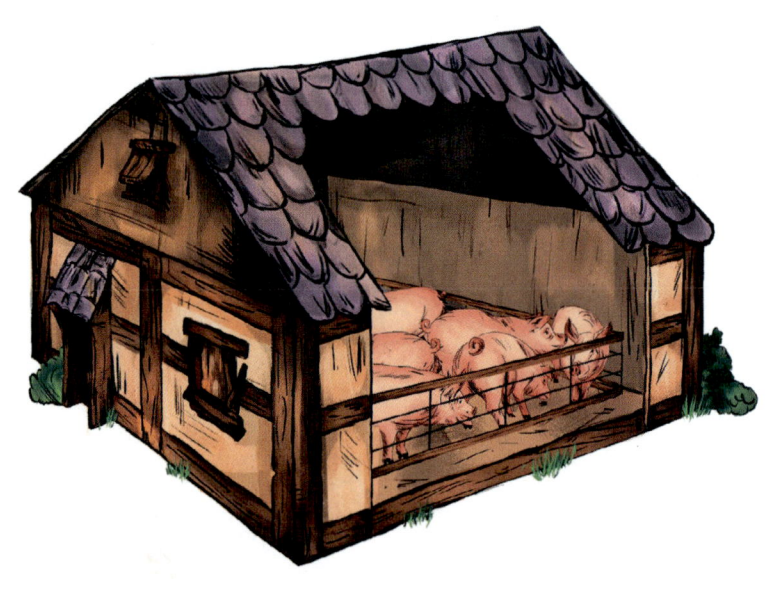

Just to give you an example of how that might feel, imagine being stuck in the middle seat in economy class on an airline between two very large people. Now imagine being stuck in that position your entire life, having to urinate and defecate on yourself. That's intolerable for even a short ride. Now imagine being stuck like that your entire life. That's what these pigs are forced to endure.

Returning to a pig's reproductive cycle, once she gives birth, the enslavement doesn't end. Instead, she is moved to another cage with her piglets, where she is once again only given enough room to stand and to lay down; she still does not have enough room to turn around. The mother pig remains with her piglets under these conditions for five weeks, until they are separated. Once separated, the mother is again artificially inseminated to repeat another brutal pregnancy cycle. When she can no longer be useful in reproducing, she is then sent to the slaughterhouse to be butchered into pieces. Given these living conditions, you can imagine that farmers have to address rampant disease among their stock. Countering disease requires more drugs and pesticides that then continue to affect the quality of the meat when it reaches your table.

It might seem that the mother pig's living situation is terrible, but it doesn't end with her and instead continues with her piglets as well. The living conditions for the piglets are no better than their mother's living conditions. Piglets are sent to group pens, where they are matured and fattened up enough to be slaughtered. These group pens house about 2000 pigs, where, on average, the pigs weigh 270 lbs. each. A single operational facility typically has three warehouses of group pens side-by-side per operation. That adds up to 6000 pigs per operation. A single pig poops about ten pounds of feces daily. For a single operation, that's 60,000 lbs. of feces per week, or roughly 2.9 million pounds of feces per year in just one facility. That's a tremendous amount of feces that pigs are living around day in, day out. Additionally, the group pens are extremely overcrowded, which further increases bacterial infections; thus, the pigs are often ill.

Understanding how much feces these pigs produce in their tight spaces help us understand the increased potential for disease and infection among the stock, which ultimately negatively affects the quality of the meat.

Confined pigs living under unnatural and stressful conditions in their own feces naturally lead to a lot of sick pigs. With rampant illness among pigs, these types of operations are only profitable and functional with the use of large amounts of antibiotics. And when I say "large," I mean very large amounts. In a typical operation, you'll see antibiotics being injected into pigs, as well as added to their food and their water. On average, you'll probably see 10-15 different antibiotics in rotation in a single operation. Can you believe it? The conditions are so poor and filthy that the pigs can't even stay alive for three months without all these drugs. That's laughable, and that's not farming. That's just disgusting and horrifying.

To make matters worse, the factory-farm pork industry relies heavily on grain to feed the pigs. And a lot of times this feed is genetically modified. The problem is that genetically-modified pig food is grown with the harmful chemical Roundup Ready. The main ingredient is glyphosate, a very toxic pesticide. Remember that you eat what your food eats, so if the pigs are eating genetically-modified food grown with harmful synthetic pesticides, you yourself will be exposed to that chemical one way or another.[1] The list of side effects from being exposed to glyphosate is endless, and that list is available in Chapter 8 GMOs.

Another problem with feeding pigs so much grain is that high-grain diets shoot the omega-6 way up, which, once again, ruins the natural balance of omega-3 to omega-6. This will cause a lot of inflammation in those who eat this type of pork.

Another little thing the factory-farm pork industry doesn't reveal is the widespread use of beta-agonist, which promotes the growth of lean muscle tissue in animals. The most popular drug in this category is Ractopamine. Banned or restricted in 160 countries, including China, Russia, and every country in the European Union, Ractopamine is still completely legal and widely used in the U.S. In fact, an estimated 60-80% of the pork produced in the U.S. and sold at the supermarket has been grown with Ractopamine.[2] When it comes to informing consumers, sure, on the packaging it states "no steroids used," but nowhere does it say "no beta-agonists used"! These are strategies used to meet standard guidelines without negatively impacting profitability and supply, but they ultimately mislead consumers--and factory-farming brands are definitely full of tricks.

GOOD CATEGORY:

FREE-RANGE PORK

Pork classified as "free-range" is a tricky category. Most of the time, what this means is that the pigs still live in a highly confined factory-farm type environment, but do have a small, concrete patio to roam outside on. This small concrete patio is usually accessible through a door which is left open for a certain number of hours daily—supposedly, if weather permits and if the planets align all at once. In reality, most of the time you typically see a lot of overcrowding in this category still, so pigs aren't allowed to express their natural behaviors.

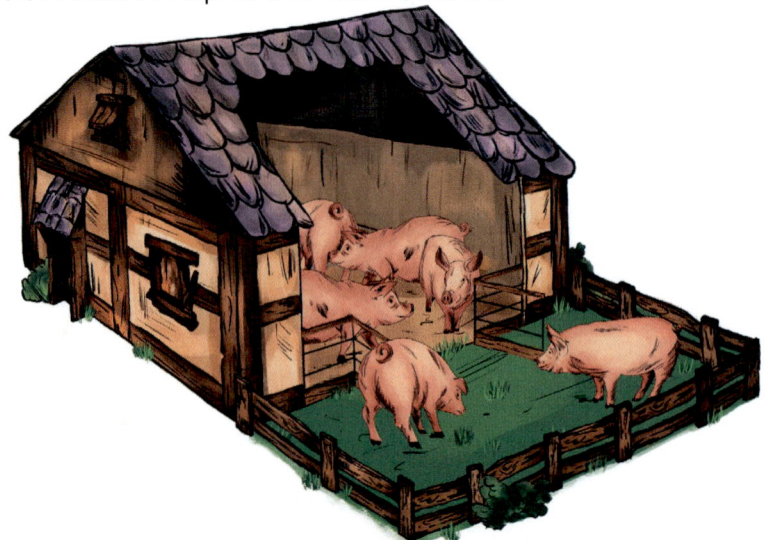

The little room they do have to move around outside is only equivalent to a small patio, so they are still unable to act like a pig. Similarly, it's likely that their main source of food is grain instead of their natural omnivore diet.

There are some respectable free-range operations. However, you typically will never see these products available at supermarkets. You'll definitely have to go to an independent farmer for this one, and once again—don't be afraid to ask for a tour. Any credible farmer will give you one.

BEST CATEGORY:

PASTURE-RAISED, ORGANIC PORK

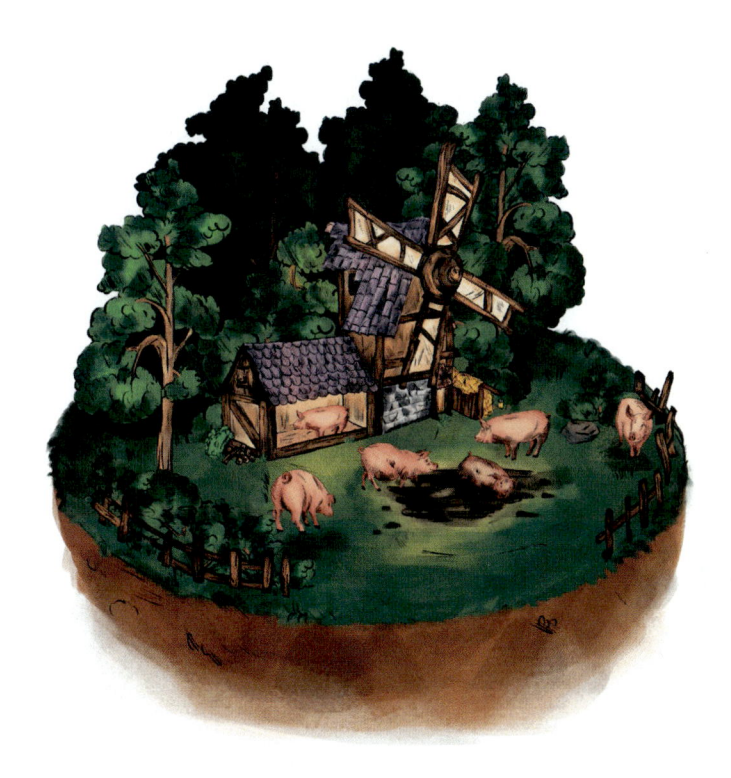

This category is as natural as they come. The female pigs in this category are never stuck in cages; they are never forced to live in their own urine and feces; and they are not injected with a ridiculous amount of antibiotics and drugs. They are also not allowed to eat genetically-modified feed.

They get to roam free 24/7 in nature with plenty of sunshine, fresh air, and plenty of room. They are allowed to root, to socialize, and to eat a natural diet of seasonal vegetables, nuts and fruits. They are allowed to play and to be entertained. It's important to recognize that these living conditions and way of life positively impact the health and quality of the meat you consume. If pigs can live healthily and naturally, then there is less need for harmful additives that make their way into our own bodies.

An example of a great pasture-raised pork operation would be www.primalpastures.com. There are many other pasture-raised pork farms out there, but I'm just using Primal Pastures as a base mark, and as a simple example of what a good pasture-raised operation looks like.

Logos to Look for

You'll definitely never find pasture-raised pork sold at the supermarket level. This is close to impossible. If you want pasture-raised pork, you will only be able to buy them from a local farmer. You can also checkout www.eatwild.com. I would avoid all pork at the supermarket, but if you have absolutely no choice, opt for products that have a "USDA Organic Certified" logo on them.

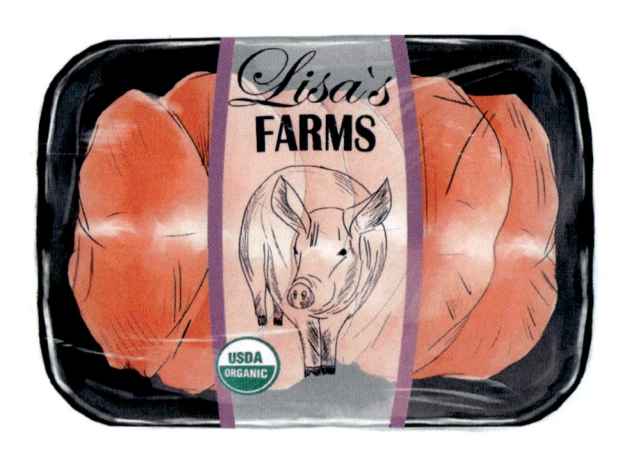

CHAPTER 8

TURKEY

Topics Covered:

- Free-range turkey doesn't mean much.
- "Vegetarian-fed" turkey isn't a good thing.
- Pasture-raised, the way it was meant to be.

WORST CATEGORY:

CAGE-FREE

There is a lot of overlap with the way chicken and turkey are produced in a factory-farm environment, which this category most definitely is. Here, about 10,000 turkeys are stuffed in a single windowless warehouse with basically no room to move. And they are forced to live under artificial light 24/7. Their beaks and claws are severed without the use of any pain killers, and they're fed a steady diet of grains, which were most definitely grown with heavy amounts of deadly, cancer-causing pesticides. Turkeys are naturally omnivores. They eat nuts, insects, worms, and various plants. They don't just eat grains! When all they're fed are grains, the natural omega-3 to omega-6 ratio, once again, is destroyed. More omega-6 to omega-3 equals more inflammation in your body and mind. And remember that all that feed is being grown with deadly pesticides. You are what your food eats. What animals are fed, gets absorbed into their tissue.[1-5]

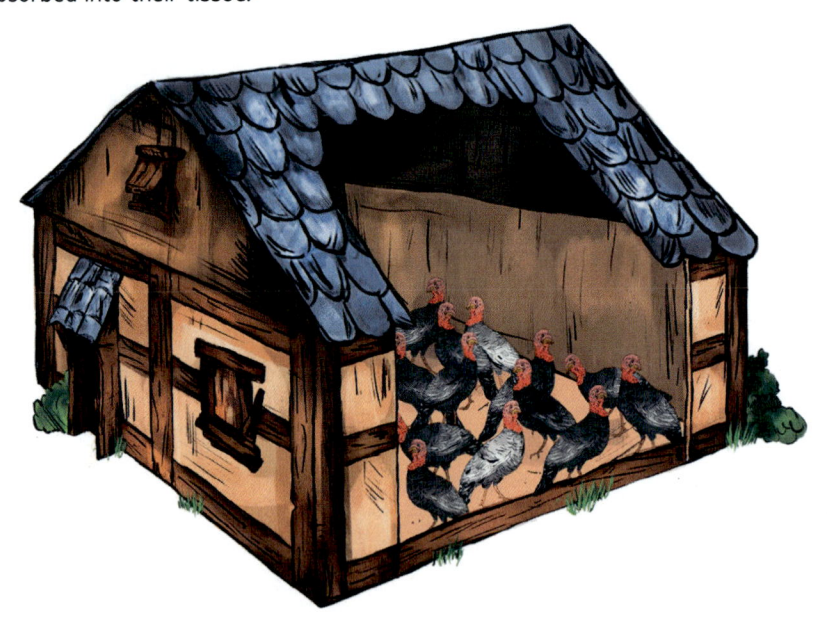

So, if the turkey you're eating is consuming pesticide-laced grain, that's going to accumulate in your body and increase your toxic load. All those chemicals are sitting and brewing in your body, and they're going to increase your chances of developing cancer and other diseases.

Another huge negative in this category is the overuse and dependence on antibiotics.

You'll see a lot of it in this category. Remember that when you stuff 10,000 large animals in a single warehouse and never let them outdoors, you're going to get a tremendous amount of fecal contamination. There are literally feces everywhere, and when combined with a very stressful environment of being crammed indoors 24/7 with 10,000 other large animals, disease breaks out. Instead of simply creating a more tolerable environment, factory farms just throw more antibiotics at the problem. Definitely stay away from this category.

GOOD CATEGORY:

FREE-RANGE

Free-range is a step in the right direction, but at the supermarket level, it doesn't really fair that much better than the category above. Here, you'll still get a tremendous amount of overcrowding where the turkeys are allowed to roam "outside" for a few hours a day—if weather permits. And by "outside," I really mean a small, fenced-off concrete patio. Few turkeys ever even bother to roam outside.

Another negative in this category is the heavy reliance on grains as a source of feed, just like the previous category. Once again, turkeys aren't vegetarians. So, if you see a "fed an all-vegetarian diet" label, even if it's organic, that's a red flag. First, that label is saying that the turkeys are not roaming freely outside. If they were roaming freely outside, they would be eating bugs too. If they're eating bugs, they can't be classified as vegetarian-fed. Secondly, if they're on a vegetarian diet, that means they're in a controlled and confined operation. They're definitely not roaming free outdoors. If they do get outdoor access, it's simply on that small concrete patio I described.

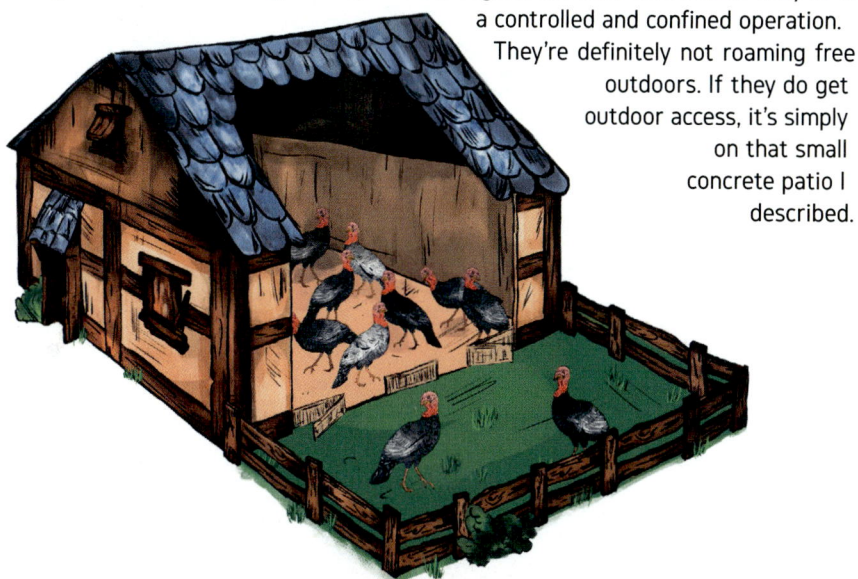

BEST CATEGORY:

PASTURE-RAISED

This is the complete opposite of what a factory-farm would produce. Here, the turkeys get to roam free outside 24/7, they get to express their natural, curious behavior, they socialize, and most importantly—they're not fed a "vegetarian diet." They eat bugs, insects, nuts, fruits, plants, and even small reptiles. All of this adds up to a far superior nutritional profile as compared to the two categories above.

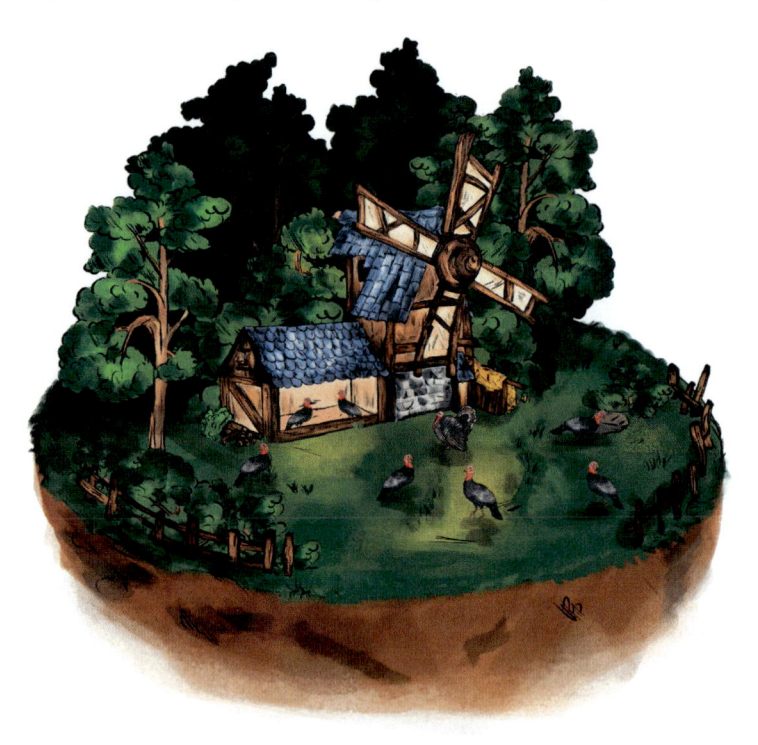

Logos to Look for

Finding pasture-raised turkey at the supermarket is going to be impossible. For this category, you're going to have to seek out a local farmer and buy it from them. If for some one-in-a-million chance your local supermarket actually does sell pasture-raised turkey, look for logos such as "USDA Organic" and "pasture-raised," "wild turkey."

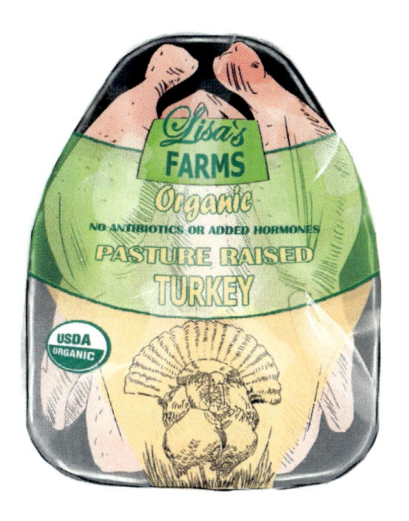

CHAPTER 9

GENETICALLY MODIFIED FOOD

Topics Covered:

- How genetically-modified food is potentially dangerous.

- How to spot genetically-modified food easily.

- Why it's important to avoid corn, soy, and canola.

- Non-GMO Project Verified and USDA Organic certifications.

With genetically-modified food, there are basically two things you have to be worried about when it comes to your health:
1. The actual genetic modification of the food.
2. The chemicals used to grow the genetically-modified food.

Genetic Modification of Food

Simply put, genetic modification is when a scientist takes a gene from one plant and embeds it into another plant through unnatural and scientific means. GMOs can only be made in the laboratory. This will never occur in nature. Some studies suggest that GMOs can cause a myriad of possible health problems ranging from damage to the gut, tumor growth, weakened immune system, stunted growth, and possible cellular damage.[1-7] Even the American Academy of Environmental Medicine urged doctors nationwide to teach their patients to follow non-genetically-modified diets.[8]

Chemicals used to grow genetically-modified food

The second danger of eating GMOs is that most GMO crops are grown with a harmful synthetic herbicide called Roundup Ready. The main ingredient in Roundup Ready is a chemical called glyphosate. Exposure to glyphosate could result in disruption to gut bacteria, cancer, chronic inflammation, decrease in testosterone, and birth defects.[9-13] In 2015, the World Health Organization classified glyphosate as a "probable carcinogenic to humans."

WORST CATEGORY:

NOT CERTIFIED

You're in danger of being exposed to GMOs if you eat corn, soy, canola, and cotton products that have not been certified as organic nor non-GMO. You can also be exposed to GMOs indirectly if you eat animals or fish that have been fed GMOs in their diet, which is a standard practice in factory farms. Typically, the main source of feed in most animal factory-farm operations is GMO corn and soy. If you eat out, you'll most likely be exposed to GMOs because a lot of restaurants, especially fast food places, use cooking oils that are made from GMOs. You might be at a restaurant eating wild-caught fish, but that fish is being cooked in GMO oils, which defeats the purpose of even eating healthy. All those healthy foods are soaking in all those toxic oils.

If you don't see anything on the label that indicates a product is non-GMO and/or organic, and you're eating corn, soy or canola, or products made from those products, your chances of being exposed to GMOs are fairly high.

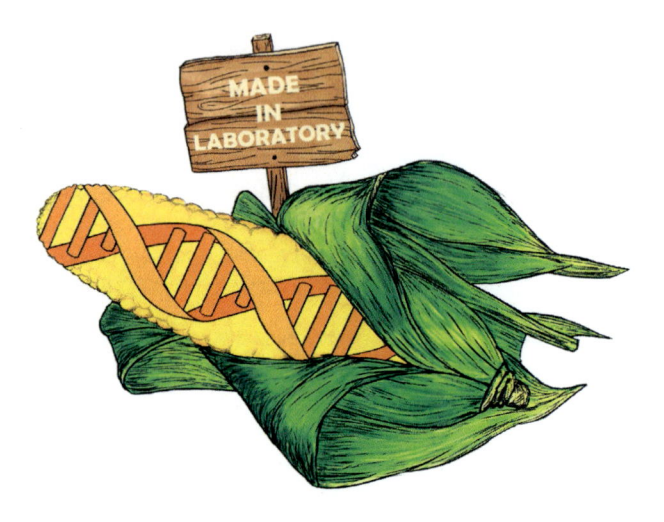

I would stay away from this category. GMOs are very sneaky. For instance, a lot of vitamin-C supplements are made from genetically-modified corn. If you look at the back of the label, you'll see "ascorbic acid." If it isn't stated that it's non-GMO, it's most likely ascorbic acid that comes from GMO corn. That's just one example of how sneaky GMOs are.

GOOD CATEGORY:

NON-GMO PROJECT VERIFIED

Your chances of being exposed to GMOs decrease if you purchase products that have been non-GMO certified by credible companies. One of my favorite certifications to look for at the supermarket level is the Non-GMO Project Verified logo. If you purchase corn, soy, canola, and cotton products that are Non-GMO Project Verified, your chances of being exposed to GMOs are reduced, but they are not at zero. Due to issues with cross-contaminations, especially in the corn industry, it's almost impossible to guarantee that the product you're purchasing is 100% GMO free.

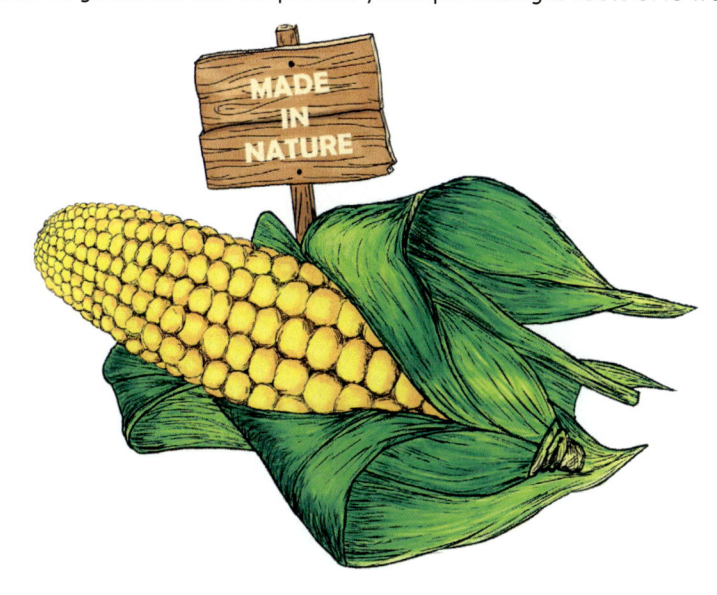

BEST CATEGORY:

NON-GMO PROJECT VERIFIED + USDA ORGANIC CERTIFIED

The absolute best way to avoid GMOs is simply to avoid corn, soy, canola, cotton, and any products made from those ingredients. This also includes animals and fish that are fed GMOs. On top of avoiding those four ingredients, I would also make sure the product is certified through the Non-GMO Project Verified certification and is USDA-Organic certified. You really do want to see both of those certifications on the label. That's going to be your absolutely best bet at avoiding exposure to GMOs.

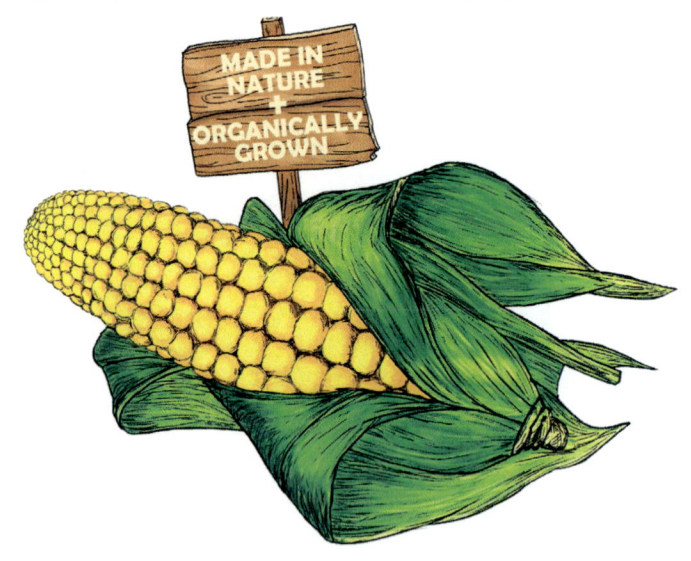

Logos to Look for

To increase your odds of avoiding GMOs, look for "Non-GMO Project Verified" certification and the logo "USDA Organic" on the same product, as shown above.

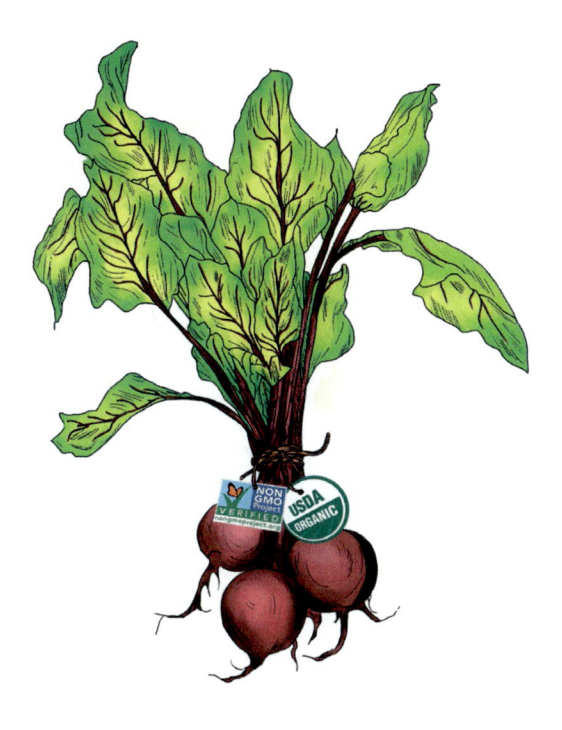

To get video instruction to this chapter, please email your receipt to etrufkin@gmail.com

CHAPTER 10

SUPPLEMENTS

Topics Covered:

- How to know you're buying a quality supplement.

- High levels of heavy metals and pesticides found in supplements.

- cGMP certification and why it's so important.

- How to find organic and non-genetically-modified supplements.

WORST CATEGORY:

GMO SUPPLEMENTS

Probably everyone and their grandmothers have taken a vitamin-C supplement at one point in their life. But what most people taking them don't know is that the vitamin-C supplement they're taking isn't coming from oranges, especially if it's from this category. I know there is a picture of an orange on the label, but in reality, most vitamin-C supplements come from genetically-modified corn and not oranges. Just look at the back of the label. You'll see "ascorbic acid." If you see "ascorbic acid," and you don't see a non-GMO certified label, or it doesn't say that it's organic, that's a dead giveaway that it's most likely made from GMO corn.

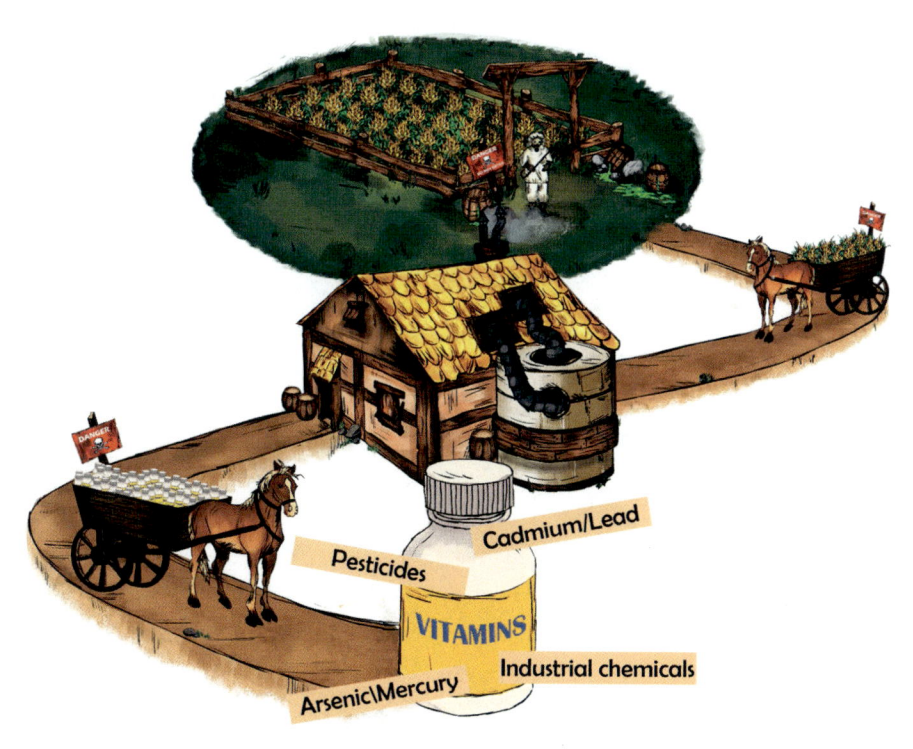

Another problem with this category is that the raw ingredients are sourced from non-organic farms: genetically-modified corn is considered non-organic. Non-organic farms use a tremendous amount of pesticides to grow crops, which often times do end up in the supplements you're taking.[1] You're taking a specific supplement to promote your health, but as a bonus you're also getting trace amounts of pesticides and heavy metals, which are detrimental to your health.[2, 3] For this reason, you want to stay away from this category. I know it's only a few bucks per bottle, but there is a reason that it's only a few bucks a bottle. Exposure to heavy metals and pesticides are very bad for your health.

GOOD CATEGORY:

NON-GMO CERTIFICATION

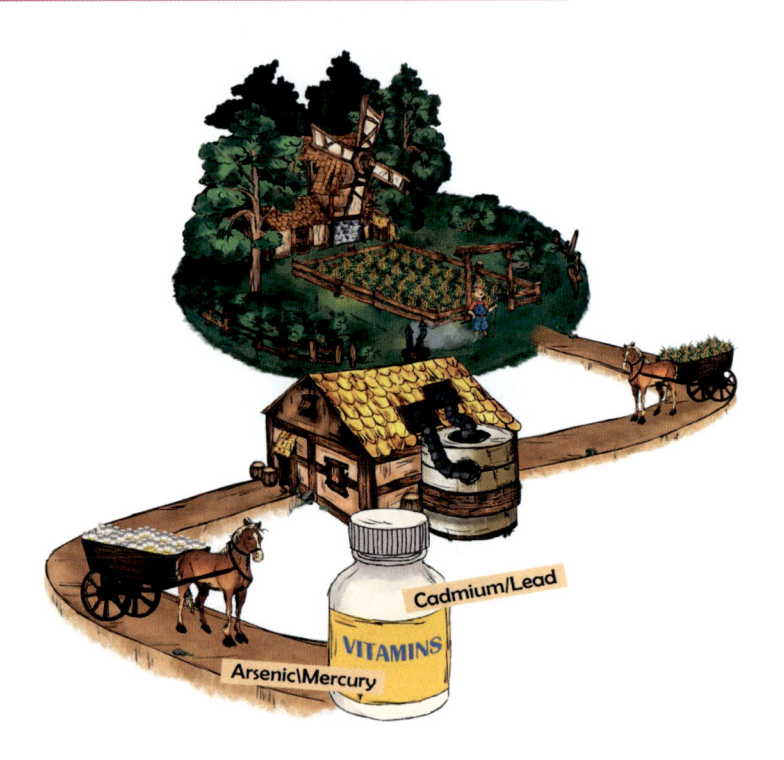

If you don't want your vitamin-C supplements to be sourced from genetically-modified corn, then make sure you see a non-GMO certification on the label. If you see a non-GMO Project Verified logo, that's going to be your best bet that the product isn't made from genetically-modified organisms. Better yet, try to look for supplements that are Non-GMO certified *and* certified organic. This will decrease your exposure to not only GMOs, but also pesticides.

SUPPLEMENTS

BEST CATEGORY:

CGMP

The best category includes everything that the good category includes (organic, non-GMO), but what's most important to consider is the way the company processes the raw ingredients, and the checks and balances they have in place to make sure their raw ingredients aren't contaminated with things like heavy metals and pesticides—which is fairly common in the supplement industry. Because contaminated supplements are so common, this is by far the most important aspect you should focus on. To check for this, go to the company's website. They should have a "quality assurance" tab. If they don't, do not buy from this company. This tab will explain the steps the company takes and the checks and balances they have in place to assure the purity of the product. Here are some aspects you want to look for. You want to make sure the company meets current Good Manufacturing Practices Guidelines for nutritional supplements. If you see that the company is certified cGMP, that's already a super huge plus. You also want to make sure the company tests every single batch for heavy metal, pesticide residue, and chemical solvents. A good example of a company that does all this would be www.poliquinstore.com.

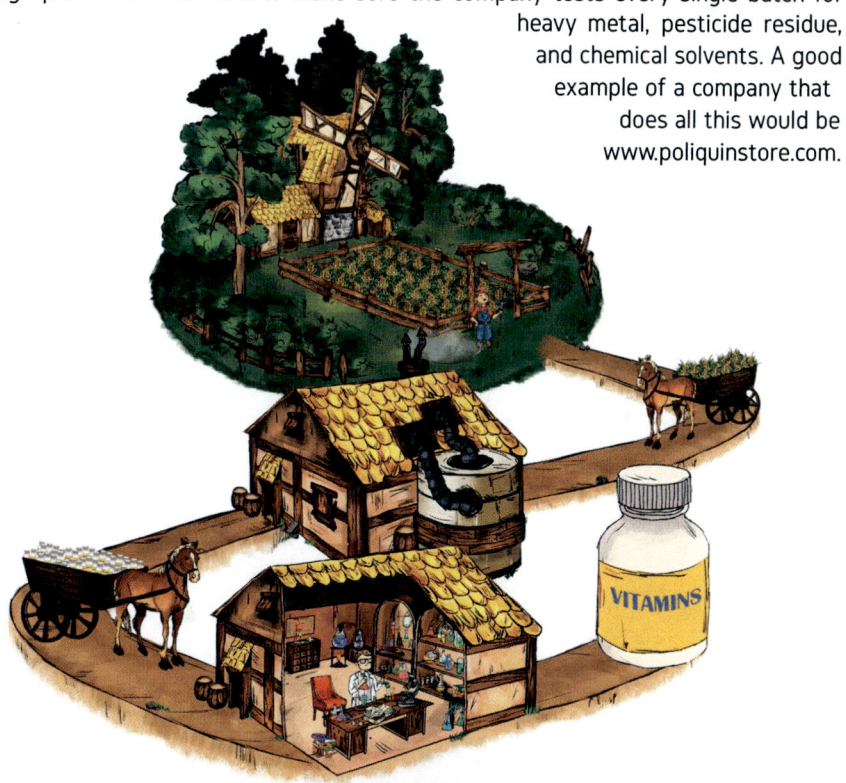

Third-Party Testing websites

Not sure if the supplements you're taking are any good—or even healthy for you? Checkout www.cleanlabelproject.org. They'll provide a detailed analyses of various supplement brands. You can also checkout www.consumerlab.com.

A word about vitamins

One thing to understand about vitamin supplements is that they're typically sold in isolated form. For example, a vitamin-C supplement is only vitamin-C. But in nature, vitamins never occur in isolation. Nowhere in nature will you see just vitamin-C alone. In an orange, for example, vitamin-C exists with other vitamins and minerals. And it's this unique vitamin complex that allows your body to recognize and properly absorb the nutrients.

In comparison, a typical vitamin-C supplement has about 1000mg of vitamin-C—that's it. However, a typical orange has about 50mg of vitamin-C and a bunch of other vitamins like vitamin-A and -B, for example. So basically, a single vitamin-C tablet of 1000mg is equivalent to eating a small bag of oranges of *just* vitamin C. However, you're not getting any vitamin-A and -B from the supplement.

That's good news you say? I'm getting so much vitamin-C. Well, it's not that simple. For our example, if you take a vitamin-C supplement but are already deficient in vitamins-A and/or -B, your body doesn't have the resources to replicate that vitamin complex as it happens in nature. And because it doesn't have those resources, it creates other nutritional deficiencies. So, you're basically solving one problem but creating two to three other problems.[4]

Now, I'm not saying isolated vitamins don't have a place in the world. What I am saying is that it will require a detailed bloodwork to know exactly which dosage you even need that vitamin in—if you even need it. For instance, if your bloodwork shows you are deficient in vitamin A, and you're only taking a vitamin-C supplement, then you might need to also take a vitamin-A supplement to create balance. You have to take all this into consideration if you want any benefits from the vitamins you take.

Logos to Look for

Look for the "USDA Organic" and "Non-GMO Project Verified" logos. Also, checkout the company's site and make sure they're compliant with cGMP standards – which most are not.

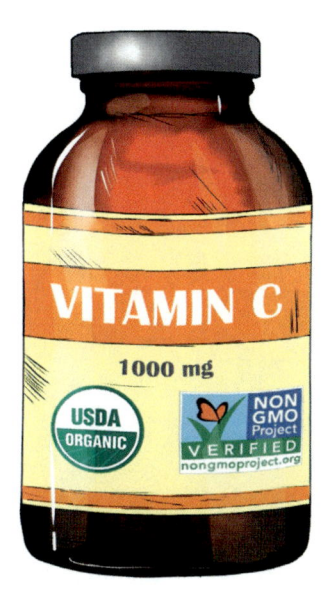

CHAPTER 11

IS ORGANIC MORE EXPENSIVE?

IS ORGANIC MORE EXPENSIVE?

One of the things I hear people say often is that organic food is just too expensive. The funny thing is that I only hear this comment from people who don't even shop organic. They just presume that organic is more expensive without doing their research. So, let's put opinions aside and see how much organic food really costs compared to factory-farmed food.

We'll compare a 2000 calorie organic diet with a 2000 calorie factory-farmed diet. The 2000 calories will be broken down into 100 grams of protein, 225 grams of carbs, and 75 grams of fat. The organic and factory-farmed food will be purchased from Sprouts in Irvine, California—a fairly high-end grocery store. You can actually find cheaper organic food such as O Organics sold at Vons, and 365 sold at Wholefoods.

FOOD GROUP	SERVING SIZE	COST OF ORGANIC	COST OF FACTORY FARM
LONG GRAIN BROWN RICE	12 OZ	$ 0.75	$ 0.68
STEEL CUT OATMEAL	8 OZ	$ 1.60	$ 1.28
WHOLE EGGS	4	$ 1.99	$ 0.92
CHICKEN	16 OZ	$ 3.00	$ 1.50
BROCCOLI	8 OZ	$ 1.24	$ 1.00
CARROTS	7 OZ	$ 0.50	$ 0.18
CUCUMBERS	HALF	$ 0.50	$ 0.25
AVOCADO	1	$ 1.50	$ 0.80
KALE	5 OZ	$ 0.46	$ 0.32
RED BELL PEPPER	7 OZ	$ 1.00	$ 0.48
TOMATO	3.5 OZ	$ 0.36	$ 0.36
TOTAL		$ 12.90	$ 7.77

So, as you can see from the chart, shopping all organic costs only $12.90/day, as compared to $7.77/day for the factory-farmed option at Sprouts, which is a higher-end grocery store. Remember that there are cheaper organic options. So, a person that's anti-organic would say something like, well, that's $5 bucks a day I can save." But are they really saving that $5? From my observation, people who don't eat organic typically eat out way more. How much does that coffee at Starbucks that they get every morning cost? $3-$5 bucks! That's $90-$150 a month on mediocre coffee that's doing nothing but giving them a short spark of energy in exchange for aged skin, sleepless nights, and chronic fatigue. A single meal at a fast-food place can run anywhere from $5-$10 bucks. With the coffee and fast-food meal, that's already $8-$15 bucks a day on unhealthy obesity-producing food. Remember that eating all organic is only $12.90/day.

Still think it's too expensive?

How about that iPhone that costs $100/month, or the fact that they might spend $100-$200 drinking, eating, and going out every weekend? How about all those costs? How about the cost of looking unhealthy day in, day out? Also, you better hope that consuming trace amounts of 10-15 pesticides on a daily basis doesn't accumulate too much in your body. Cancer can be extremely costly. I know a person that spent over a million trying to fight off cancer, and still died from it. How about that cost? Eating organic doesn't seem too expensive now, does it?

… CHAPTER 12

BIOMAGNIFICATION AND TOXIC LOAD

BIOMAGNIFICATION AND TOXIC LOAD

The important take-away from why you should avoid factory-farmed food is the principal of biomagnification. Toxicity builds up and gets more lethal the higher it goes up the food chain. And now, humans are at the top of the chain.

Here is how it works

Let's say some pesticides are sprayed on corn, and it leaves pesticide residue on the outside and inside the tissue of the corn. Let's also say one unit of corn has ten units of pesticides. Thus, the toxic load of a single piece of corn is ten units, just as an example.

Now, once the corn is harvested, it's fed to chicken at a factory-farm. A chicken eats ten pieces of corn during its entire life. Each piece of corn has ten units of pesticides, so the chicken in question has been exposed to a hundred units of pesticides that have built up in the chicken's body. The toxic load of a single chicken is thus a hundred units.

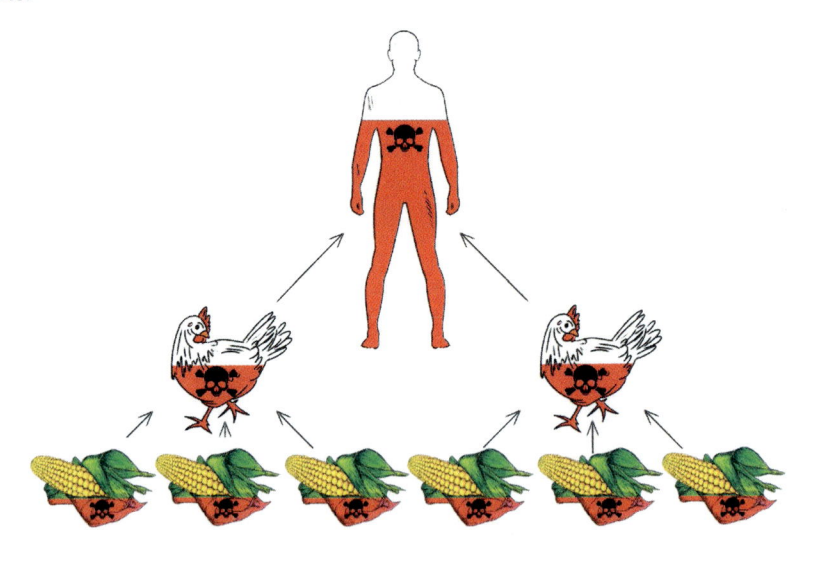

Once the chicken is slaughtered, it ends up in the grocery store where you end up buying it. Let's say during a span of the entire year, you eat about thirty chickens. Each chicken has a toxic load of a hundred units. Your toxic load from eating the thirty chickens is 3000 units. Thus, because of the principal of biomagnification, your toxic load is the highest at 3000 units.

But it doesn't stop there. You're not only eating chicken. On a weekly basis, you're also eating other meats, vegetables, fruits, soda, coffee, and a myriad of other food. If all of these foods are sourced from a factory-farmed operation, the toxic load in your body is going to be overwhelming. The higher the toxic load is in your body, the more body fat your body will create to store all those toxins. Then all those toxins just end up sitting there, brewing, and making you sick, overweight, unhealthy, and haggard looking. And results speak for themselves. Just step outside anywhere in America, which is highly dependent on factory-farmed food, and the large majority of people you will run into are full of mental and physical pain, and full of disease and obesity. Follow in their footsteps and you get their results.

Chapter 1. Vegetables and Fruits

1. U.S. Department of Agriculture (2016). Pesticide Data Program: Annual Summary, Calendar Year 2015 [Data file]. Retrieved from https://www.ams.usda.gov/sites/default/files/media/2015PDPAnnualSummary.pdf
2. Curl, C., Fenske, R., & Elgethun, K. (2003). Organophosphorus pesticide exposure of urban and suburban preschool children with organic and conventional diets. Environmental Health Perspectives, 111(3), 377-382. Retrieved from https://www.ncbi.nlm.nih.gov/pubmed/12611667
3. Marrs, C. (2014). Is it time to include inactive ingredients in chemical safety testing? Hormones Matter, February 4, 2014. Retrieved from http://www.hormonesmatter.com/chemical-safety-testing-adjuvants/.
4. Richard, S., Moslemi, S., Sipahutar, H., Benachour, N., & Seralini, GE. (2005). Differential effects of glyphosate and roundup on human placental cells and aromatase. Environmental Health Perspectives, 113(6), 716-720. Retrieved from https://www.ncbi.nlm.nih.gov/pmc/articles/PMC1257596/
5. Colborn, T. (2005) A Case for revisiting the safety of pesticides: a closer look at neurodevelopment. Environmental Health Perspectives, 114(1), 10-17. Retrieved from https://www.ncbi.nlm.nih.gov/pmc/articles/PMC1332649/
6. Houlihan, J., Kropp, T., Wiles, R., Sean, G., & Campbell, C. (2005). BodyBurden: The pollution in newborns: a benchmark investigation of industrial chemicals, pollutants, and pesticides in human umbilical cord blood [PDF file]. Retrieved from https://assets.ctfassets.net/t0qcl9kymnlu/2GVUmYpZCgu6iuSiKEUY4m/9ccbb2938066649259c634806957d499/Body_Burden_in_Newborns.pdf
7. Lifetime risk of developing or dying from cancer. (January 4, 2018). Retrieved from https://www.cancer.org/cancer/cancer-basics/lifetime-probability-of-developing-or-dying-from-cancer.html
8. Thongprakaisang, S., Thiantanawat, A., Rangkadilok, N., Suriyo, T., & Satayavivad, J. (2013). Glyphosate induces human breast cancer cells growth via estrogen receptors. Food and Chemical Toxicology: An International Journal Published for the British Industrial Biological Research Association. 59. doi:10.1016/j.fct.2013.05.057.

Chapter 2. Water

1. 1. Fox, M., (YEAR). Healthy Water for a Longer Life: A Nutritionist look at Drinking Water. Title of Book, page range.

Chapter 3. Eggs

1. Karsten, H., Patterson, P., Stout, R., & Crews, G. (2010). Vitamins A, E and fatty acid composition of the eggs of caged hens and pastured hens. Renewable Agriculture and Food Systems, 25(1), 45-54. doi:10.1017/S1742170509990214
2. Nutritional benefits of higher welfare animal products (2012). [PDF file]. Retrieved from https://www.compassioninfoodbusiness.commedia/5234769/Nutritional-benefits-of-higher-welfare-animal-products-June-2012.pdf
3. Simopoulos, A. P. (2008). The importance of the omega-6/omega-3 fatty acid ratio in cardiovascular disease and other chronic diseases. Experimental Biology and Medicine, 233(6), 674–688. Retrieved from https://doi.org/10.3181/0711-MR-311
4. Hunter P. (2012). The inflammation theory of disease. The growing realization that chronic inflammation is crucial in many diseases opens new avenues for treatment. EMBO reports, 13(11), 968-70. Retrieved from https://www.ncbi.nlm.nih.gov/pmc/articles/PMC3492709/

Chapter 4. Chicken

1. Altekruse, S. F., Berrang, M. E., Marks, H., Patel, B., Shaw, W. K., Saini, P., Bennett, P. A., & Bailey, J. S. (2009). Enumeration of Escherichia coli cells on chicken carcasses as a potential measure of microbial process control in a random selection of slaughter establishments in the United States. Applied and Environmental Microbiology, 75(11), 3522-7. Retrieved from https://www.ncbi.nlm.nih.gov/pmc/articles/PMC2687290/
2. Mellon, M., Benbrook, C., & Benbrook, K.L., (2001). Hoggin it!: estimates of antimicrobial abuse in livestock. Union of Concerned Scientists: Science for a Healthy Planet and Safer World. [PDF file] Retrieved from https://www.ucsusa.org/food_and_agriculture/our-failing-food-system/industrial-agriculture/hogging-it-estimates-of.html#.XGYzqy3MyqB
3. Waters, A.E., Contente-Cuomo, T., Buchhagen, J., Liu, C., Watson, L., Pearce, K., . . . Price, L.B., (2011). Multidrug-Resistant Staphylococcus aureus in US Meat and Poultry. Clinical Infectious Diseases 52(10), 1227–1230. Retrieved from https://doi.org/10.1093/cid/cir181
4. Researchers find evidence of banned antibiotics in poultry products. (2012). Retrieved from https://www.jhsph.edu/news/news-releases/2012/feather-meal-clf.html

Chapter 5. Beef

1. Handa, Y., Fujita, H., Honma, H., Minakami, R., (2009). Estrogen concentrations in beef and human hormone-dependent cancers. Annals of Oncology, 20(9), 1610-1611. Retrieved from https://doi.org/10.1093/annonc/mdp381
2. Prentice, G. (April 19, 2011). Got milk? What about drugs? Retrieved from https://

www.inlander.com/spokane/got-milk-what-about-drugs/Content?oid=2134801
3. Duckett, S.K., Neel, J.P.S., Fontenot, J.P., & Clapham, W.M., (2014). Effects of winter stocker growth rate and finishing system on: III. Tissue proximate, fatty acid, vitamin, and cholesterol content. [PDF file]. Retrieved from https://pdfs.semanticscholar.org/a776/a3788cf06053c8d38cb4766d1846f22bfe9a.pdf?_ga=2.238683589.472985812.1545352566-833198508.1545352566
4. Ponnampalam, E.N., Mann, N.J., Sinclair, A.J., (2006). Effect of feeding systems on omega-3 fatty acids, conjugated linoleic acid and trans fatty acids in Australian beef cuts: potential impact on human health. Asia Pac J Clin Nutr, 15(1), 21-29. Retrieved from http://citeseerx.ist.psu.edu/viewdoc/download?doi=10.1.1.563.621&rep=rep1&type=pdf

Chapter 6. Fish

1. Ibrahim, M. M., Fjære, E., Lock, E. J., Naville, D., Amlund, H., Meugnier, E., Le Magueresse Battistoni, B., Frøyland, L., Madsen, L., Jessen, N., Lund, S., Vidal, H., ... Ruzzin, J. (2011). Chronic consumption of farmed salmon containing persistent organic pollutants causes insulin resistance and obesity in mice. PloS one, 6(9), e25170. Retrieved from https://www.ncbi.nlm.nih.gov/pmc/articles/PMC3179488/
2. Lundebye, A.K., Hove, H., Mage, A., Bohne, V.J.B., & Hamre, K., (2010). Levels of synthetic antioxidant (ethoxyquin, butylated hydroxytoluene and butylated hydroxyanisole) in fish feed and commercially farmed fish. Food Additives & Contaminants: Part A, 27(12), 1652-1657. Retrieved from https://doi.org/10.1080/19440049.2010.508195
3. Ortelli, D., Cognard, E., Stuab-Sporn, A., & Edder, P., (2011). Proceedings from 5th International Symposium: Recent Advances in Food Analysis. Prague, Czech Republic.
4. Kaneko, J.J., & Ralston, N.V.C., (2007) Biol Trace Elem Res, 119(3), 242-254. Retrieved from https://doi.org/10.1007/s12011-007-8004-8
5. Parizek, O.J., (1967). The Protective effect of small amounts of selenite in sublimate intoxication. Experientia, 23(2), 142-143. Retrieved from https://www.ncbi.nlm.nih.gov/pubmed/6032113?report=docsum

Chapter 7. Pork

1. Sharma, R., Damgaard, D., Alexander, T.W., Dungan, M.E.R., Aalhus, J.L., Stanford, K., & McAllister, T.A. (2006). J. Agric. Food Chem, 54(5), 1699-1709. Retrievied from https://www.ncbi.nlm.nih.gov/m/pubmed/16506822/?i=4&from=/12817492/related6506822/?i=4&from=/12817492/related
2. Pork chops and ground pork contaminated with bacteria. (January 2013). Retrieved from https://www.consumerreports.org/cro/magazine/2013/01/what-s-in-that-pork/index.htm

Chapter 8. GMOs

1. Seralini, G.E., Clair, E., Mesnage, R., Gress, S., Defarge, N., Malatesta, M., Hennequin, D., & de Vendomois, J.S., (2012). Long term toxicity of a Roundup herbicide and a Roundup-tolerant genetically modified maize. Food Chem Toxicol, 50(11), 4221-4231. Retrieved from https://www.ncbi.nlm.nih.gov/pubmed/22999595
2. Smith, J., (December 31, 2010). Throwing biotech lies at tomatoes – part 1: killer tomatoes. Huff Post. Retrieved from https://www.huffingtonpost.com/jeffrey-smith/throwing-biotech-lies-at_b_803139.html
3. Mesnage, R., Clair, E., Gress, S., Then, C., Székács, A., & Séralini, G., (2013). Cytotoxicity on human cells of Cry1Ab and Cry1Ac Bt insecticidal toxins alone or with a glyphosate-based herbicide. J. Appl. Toxicol., 33: 695-699. doi:10.1002/jat.2712
4. Mezzomo, B.P., Miranda-Vilela, A.L., Freire, I.S., Barbosa, D.C.P., Portilho, F.A., et al. (2013). Hematotoxicity of Bacillus thuringiensis as Spore-crystal Strains Cry1Aa, Cry1Ab, Cry1Ac or Cry2Aa in Swiss Albino Mice. J Hematol Thromb Dis, 1(1). 1-9. doi: 10.4172/2329-8790.1000104
5. Ermakova, I., (n.d.). Influence of genetically modified soya on the birth-weight and survival of rat pups. Greenpeace, 41-47. Retrieved from http://somloquesembrem.org/wp-content/uploads/2013/01/Ermakovasoja.pdf
6. Key FDA documents revealing the abnormal risks in genetically engineered foods—and flaws with how agency made its policy. Alliance for Bio-Integrity, Retrieved from https://www.omicsonline.org/open-access/hematotoxicity-of-bacillus-thuringiensis-as-spore-crystal-strains-cry1aa-cry1ab-cry1ac-or-cry2aa-in-swiss-albino-mice-2329-8790.1000104.pdf?url=JHTD/JHTD-1-104.pdf
7. Dean, A., & Armstrong, J., (May 8, 2009). Genetically modified foods. American Academy of Environmental Medicine. Retrieved from https://www.aaemonline.org/gmo.php
8. Dean, A., & Armstrong, J., (May 8, 2009). Genetically modified foods. American Academy of Environmental Medicine. Retrieved from https://www.aaemonline.org/gmo.php
9. Shehata, A.A., Schrödl, W., Aldin, A.A. et al., (2013) Curr Microbiol, 66(350). https://doi.org/10.1007/s00284-012-0277-2
10. Samsel, A., & Seneff, S., (2013). Glyphosate's Suppression of Cytochrome P450 Enzymes and Amino Acid Biosynthesis by the Gut Microbiome: Pathways to Modern Diseases. Entropy 15, 1416-1463. Retrieved from https://www.mdpi.com/1099-4300/15/4/1416
11. Clair, E., Mesnage, R., Travert, C., & Seralini, G.E., (March 2012). A glyphosate-based herbicide induces necrosis and apoptosis in mature rat testicular cells in vitro, and testosterone decrease at lower levels. Toxicology in Vitro, 26(2), 269-279. Retrieved from https://www.sciencedirect.com/science/article/pii/S0887233311003341?via%3Dihub

12. Krüger, M., Schrödl, W., Pedersen, Ib., Schledorn, P., & Shehata, AA., (2014). Detection of Glyphosate in Malformed Piglets. J Environ Anal. Toxicol 4(230). doi: 10.4172/2161-0525.1000230
13. Swanson, N.L., Leu, A., Abrahamson, J., & Wallet, B., (2014). Genetically engineered crops, glyphosate and the deterioration of health in the United States of America. Journal of Organic Systems, 9(2). Retrieved from http://www.organic-systems.org/journal/92/abstracts/Swanson-et-al.html

Chapter 9. Turkey

1. Giuliana, M., Dazzi, G., Campanini, G., & Maggi, E., (1979). Organochlorine pesticide residues in meat of various species. Elsevier, 4(2), 157-166. Retrieved from https://www.sciencedirect.com/science/article/abs/pii/030917408090039X?via%3Dihub
2. Ahmad, S., Rehman, R., Haider, S., Batool, Z., Ahmed, F., Ahmed, S.B., Perveen, T., Rafiq, S., Sadir, S., & Shahzad, S., (2018). Quantitative and qualitative assessment of additives present in broiler chicken feed and meat and their implications for human health. J Pak Med Assoc, 68(6), 876-881. Retrieved from https://www.ncbi.nlm.nih.gov/pubmed/30325904
3. Panseri, S., Biondi, P.A., Vigo, D., Communod, R., & Chiesa, L. M., (January 16th 2013). Occurrence of Organochlorine Pesticides Residues in Animal Feed and Fatty Bovine Tissue, Food Industry. IntechOpen, DOI: 10.5772/54182. Available from: https://www.intechopen.com/books/food-industry/occurrence-of-organochlorine-pesticides-residues-in-animal-feed-and-fatty-bovine-tissue
4. Bedi, J.S., Gill, J.P.S., Kuar, P., & Aulakh, R.S., (January 2018). Pesticide residues in milk and their relationship with pesticide contamination of feedstuffs supplied to dairy cattle in Punjab (India), Journal of Animal and Feed Sciences, 27(1), 18-25. Retrieved from http://www.jafs.com.pl/Pesticide-residues-in-milk-and-their-relationship-with-pesticide-contamination-of,82623,0,2.html
5. Mahugija, J.A.M., Chibura, P.E., & Lugwisha, E.H.J., (2017). Residues of pesticides and metabolites in chicken kidney, liver and muscle samples from poultry farms in Dar es Salaam and Pwani, Tanzania, Chemosphere, 193, 869-874. Retrieved from https://www.ncbi.nlm.nih.gov/pubmed/29874761

Chapter 10. Supplements

1. 1Chen, Y., Lopez S., Hayward, DG., Park, H.Y., Wong, J.W., Kim, S.S., Wan, J., Reddy, R.M., Quinn, D.J., and Steiniger, D., (2016). Determination of Multiresidue Pesticides in Botanical Dietary Supplements Using Gas Chromatography-Triple-Quadrupole Mass Spectrometry (GC-MS/MS). J Agric Food Chem., 64(31), 6125-32. Retrieved from https://www.ncbi.nlm.nih.gov/pubmed/27101866
2. Wong, J.W., Wirtz, M.S., Hennessy, M.K., Schenck, F.J., Krynitsky, A.J. & Capar, S.G. (2006). Pesticides in botanical dietary supplements. Acta Hortic, 720, 113-

128. Retrieved from https://doi.org/10.17660/ActaHortic.2006.720.11
3. Schwalfenberg, G., Rodushkin, I., & Genuis, S. J. (2018). Heavy metal contamination of prenatal vitamins. Toxicology reports, 5, 390-395. doi:10.1016/j.toxrep.2018.02.015
4. Chek, P., (2013). What is organics? Part 4: The Vitamin Complex. Retrieved from https://www.paulcheksblog.com/what-is-organics-part-4-the-vitamin-complex/

Made in the USA
Middletown, DE
15 January 2020